REMOVABLE PARTIAL PROSTHODONTICS:

a case-orientated manual of treatment planning

Dr Sybille K Lechner
Department of Prosthodontics, The Dental School, University of Sydney,
Sydney, NSW 2000, Australia

Professor A R MacGregor
Department of Prosthodontics, Glasgow Dental School and Hospital,
Glasgow, Scotland

⋈ Wolfe

Copyright © 1994 Mosby–Year Book Europe Limited

Published in 1994 by Wolfe Publishing, an imprint of Mosby–Year Book Europe Limited

Printed and bound in Great Britain by BPCC Hazell Books Ltd

ISBN 0 7234 1960 4

For full details of all Mosby–Year Book Europe Limited titles please write to Mosby–Year Book Europe Limited, Lynton House, 7–12 Tavistock Square, London WC1H 9LB, England.

A CIP catalogue record for this book is available from the British Library.

Library of Congress Cataloging-in-Publication Data
MacGregor, A. Roy (Alastair Roy)
    Removable partial prosthodontics: a case oriented manual of
treatment / Alastair Roy MacGregor, Sybille K. Lechner.
    p.   cm.
    Includes bibliographical references.
    ISBN 0-7234-1960-4
    1. Partial dentures. Removable—Design and construction.
2. Partial dentures, removable—Design and construction—Case
studies.   I. Lechner, S. K.   II. Title.
    [DNLM: 1. Denture, Partial, Removable.   2. Patient Care Planning.
3. Periodontal Diseases—therapy—case studies.   WU 515 M147n 1993]
RK665.M23   1993
617.6'92—dc20
DNLM/DLC
for Library of Congress   93-2006
                                                                        CIP

Contents

Introduction

There are many excellent textbooks that deal with the clinical and laboratory aspects of removable partial dentures. From these one can learn the finer points of partial denture theory and practice. It is often difficult, however, for dental students and practitioners to condense such a huge amount of information into a workable treatment plan for a patient.

There are also those textbooks which seem to oversimplify and which present standardised designs for various combinations of tooth loss without regard to the infinite variety possible, such as differences among the patients themselves, dental history, biological background, tooth form and position, occlusion, and so on.

For these reasons we feel there is a need for something to bridge the gap between a detailed text and such a 'design by rote' approach.

In presenting this manual we assume that you have a working knowledge of the physiology and pathology of the oral cavity. We also assume that you are reasonably familiar with partial denture components, their functions, dimensions and variations, and that you have in front of you the medical and dental history, examination charts, radiographs and articulated, surveyed study casts of your patient.

Where do you go from here? How do you channel all the information into a cohesive, workable treatment plan and denture design for the patient you are treating?

We have tried to present a step-by-step, rational approach, describing basic principles and simple, reliable techniques which will make working with the partially edentulous patient both predictable and successful.

We hope we have succeeded and that you find this manual helpful.

Acknowledgements

Our grateful thanks are due to Pat Hercus and Rebecca Granger for secretarial help in arranging, typing and editing the script.

Ann Hughes produced most of the line drawings from originals supplied by one of us (S.K.L.); the casts were assembled and produced by Michael Broad; the photographs were made by David Woodward, John Davies and Kay Shepherd; to all these colleagues, and others who have helped in many ways, we are sincerely grateful.

I (S.K.L.) would like to thank Campbell H Graham, who first made me realise that the oral cavity is attached to a patient, and that patients are people. I would also like to thank Cyril J Thomas for some excellent ideas, and I am particularly grateful to Graham A Thomas, who spent much time arguing with me about patients and their problems, and so kept me from becoming complacent.

Tooth Notation

This book uses the FDI two-digit system of tooth notation. The first digit of each pair of numbers indicates the quadrant. The second digit indicates the tooth within that quadrant (Fig **1**).

Quadrants:

1 maxillary right   3 mandibular left
2 maxillary left   4 mandibular right

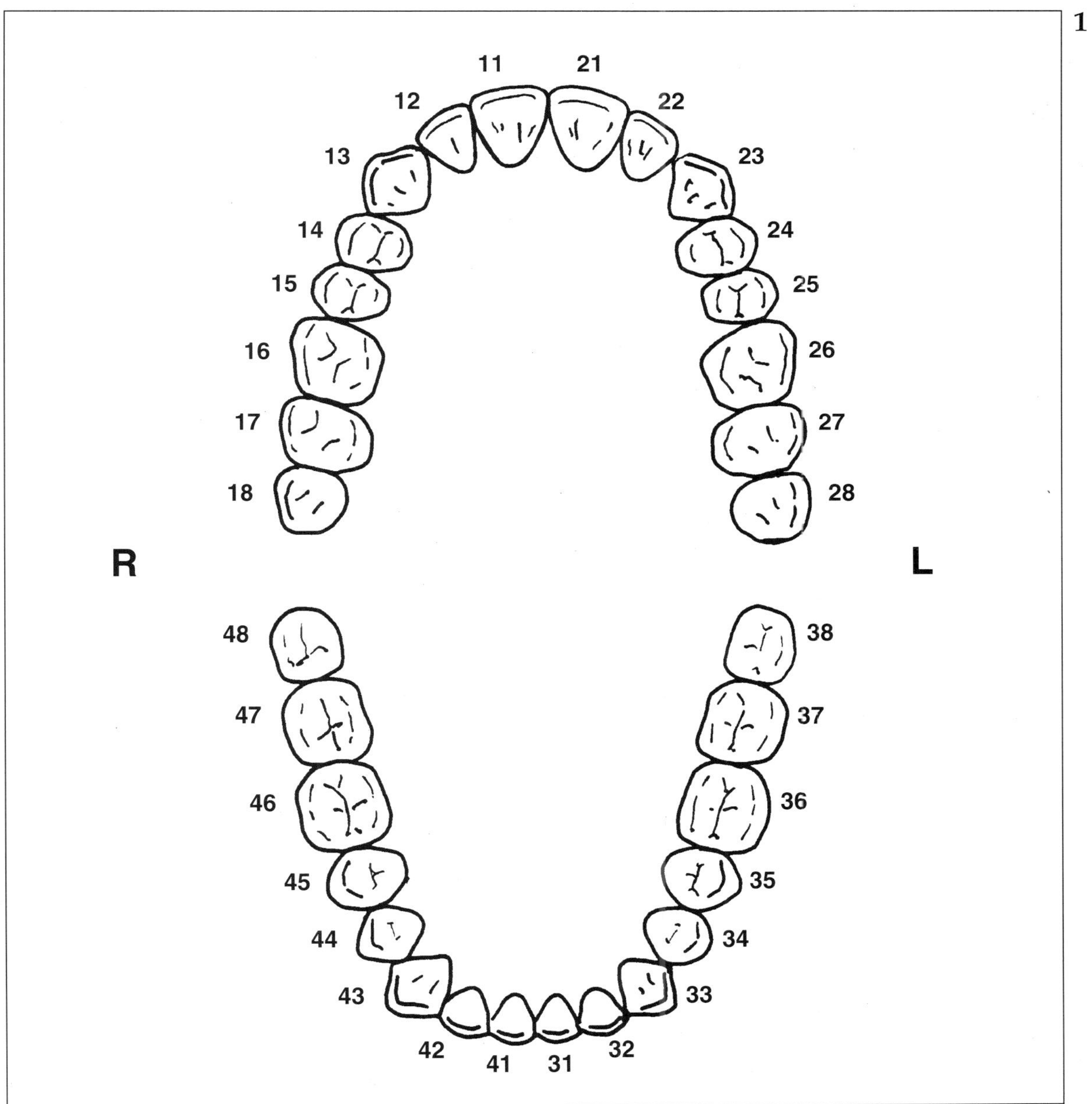

Fig **1** Tooth notation.

Glossary of Abbreviations

AR	additional retention
C overdenture	complete overdenture
c/o	complaining of
DEB	distal extension base
FPD	fixed partial denture (bridge)
GP	guide plane
IR	indirect retention
o/e	on examination
OVD	occlusal vertical dimension
PDH	past dental history
PMH	past medical history
R	retainer
RP overdenture	removable partial overdenture
RPD	removable partial denture
TSL	tooth surface loss

Tooth surfaces:

(M)	mesial	(L)	lingual	(DL)	distolingual
(D)	distal	(ML)	mesiolingual	(DB)	distobuccal
(B)	buccal	(MB)	mesiobuccal	(DP)	distopalatal
(P)	palatal	(MP)	mesiopalatal		

PART I

1 Treatment Planning

After taking the medical and dental history and examining the patient, you should be thoroughly familiar with his/her needs and wants. By now you should also know the patient as a person and why he/she wants a new denture—this is usually to improve either aesthetics or masticatory efficiency.

You will also know whether a removable partial denture (RPD) will help the *dental condition* of your patient. This is related to:

- Restoration of the occlusion.
- Space maintenance; that is, prevention of overeruption, tipping and/or tilting of remaining teeth.
- More favourable load distribution.

All this information will allow you to decide:

- Whether to make an RPD.
- What kind of RPD to design.
- Which edentulous areas to restore.

Should you make an RPD?

Would a fixed restoration be better for this patient? Make your decision after considering all the indications and contra-indications for fixed prosthodontics.

You may decide to make neither a fixed nor a removable appliance. Such a decision could be made where the patient is quite content with his/her appearance and masticatory function (despite the fact that large edentulous areas exist) and tooth migration has been minimal, even though teeth were lost some time ago.

Another situation where you would not make a denture at all is where oral hygiene is poor and the patient's dental awareness is limited, so that an RPD becomes a periodontal hazard.

What kind of RPD should you make?

Should you make a *definitive* denture (usually cobalt-chromium) or a *transitional* denture (usually acrylic resin)? A transitional RPD could be a diagnostic denture made to test the effects of preliminary treatment of changes to the occlusion, before carrying out more permanent treatment.

A transitional RPD could also be used for a patient who will probably not be able to maintain the existing dentition for much longer. For example, if the teeth are periodontally involved with a poor prognosis, a transitional denture can slowly be converted to a complete denture by adding teeth to it as the dentition is depleted.

Acrylic dentures worn over a long period of time tend to be destructive because they must cover a larger area for adequate strength. Many are also completely mucosa supported, which is an especial problem in the mandible, where the available denture-bearing area is much smaller than in the maxilla.

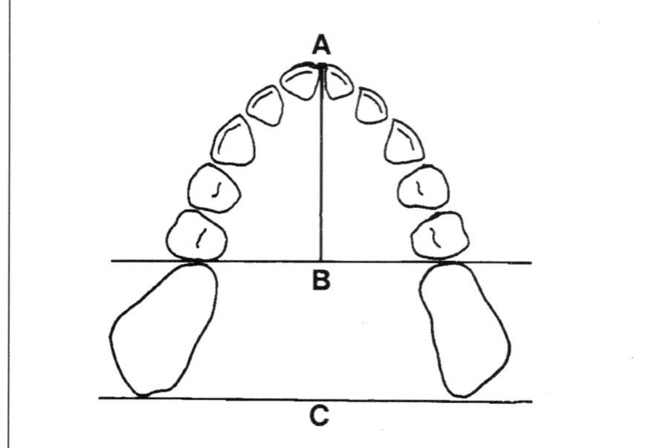

Fig 2 Curved arch. AB is equal to or greater than BC. Posterior tooth replacement is probably not necessary.

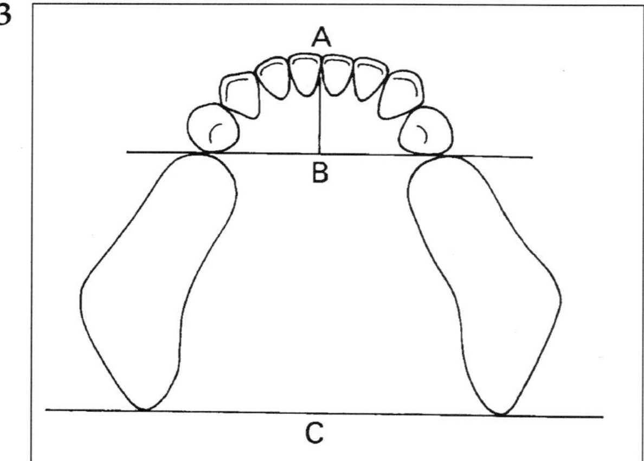

Fig 3 Flattened arch. AB is less than BC. Posterior tooth replacement is probably necessary.

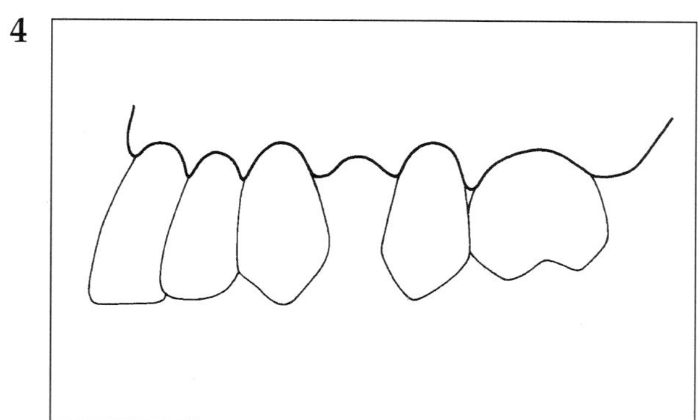

Fig 4 23 and 25 have tilted into the space left by missing 24, making restoration difficult.

Which edentulous areas should you restore?

Restore only:

- Those edentulous areas which the *patient* wants restored for aesthetics or function.
- Those areas which are needed to restore or preserve occlusal integrity.

Which edentulous areas should you *not* restore?

Try to avoid *distal extension bases* (DEBs). They have a limited success rate and are far more troublesome than tooth-bounded bases. In the absence of symptoms, occlusal support is rarely needed distal to the second premolar area as long as the arch is curved like a catenary (Figs 2, 3).

Some reasons for restoring edentulous areas distal to the second premolar might be:

- To improve aesthetics—some patients feel that their cheeks will cave in if the posterior part of the mouth is not restored.
- To provide stability for an opposing complete denture.
- To prevent overeruption of opposing natural teeth. DEBs are not very efficient in this regard as the underlying mucosa may become sore and in need of relief if the opposing teeth continue to erupt. If an RPD is needed in the opposing jaw, it is more effective to place an occlusal rest on the 'at risk' tooth itself than to try to stop overeruption with an opposing DEB.

Avoid restoring *very small edentulous areas*. Often the abutment teeth on either side of a single lost tooth drift or tilt into the space making restoration very difficult (Fig 4).

Before you decide *not* to restore such a space, discuss it with your patient. This space may be the very reason that he/she really wants treatment. You may want to consider a fixed restoration in such cases. On the other hand, the patient may not care about that space and not restoring it could make the denture design much simpler.

Having decided on these important points:

- whether to make an RPD at all
- what kind of RPD to make
- which edentulous areas to restore

you can begin to design the denture in line with the design principles outlined in Chapter 2.

2 Design Principles

These are basic design principles only and presuppose a knowledge of individual denture components, their shape, dimensions and general uses, obtained from textbooks and other literature (see Bibliography).

Important points to remember for all designs:

- Existing denture(s).
- Tissue preservation.
- Occlusal integrity.
- Oral hygiene and maintenance.
- Resistance to various forces.

Existing denture(s)

Note the details of any RPD the patient is already wearing. It will tell you what the patient has or has not been able to cope with in the past and what response this patient's tissues have had to various denture components. Your design could well copy non-traumatic elements of the existing design.

Tissue preservation

In 1952 De Van wrote: 'Our objective should be the perpetual preservation of what remains rather than the meticulous restoration of what is missing.' It has been shown from a number of partial denture surveys (Anderson and Lammie, 1952; Anderson and Bates, 1959; Brill *et al.*, 1977; Lechner, 1985*b*; Seemann, 1963) that an RPD has great potential to damage the oral tissues. Make sure that your partial denture causes as little damage as possible:

- Place it in the healthy mouth of a patient who will maintain good oral hygiene.
- Cover as little tooth and mucosa as is consistent with adequate load distribution and other mechanical factors. If possible leave gingival margins uncovered, but do not get caught in a 'small window' situation as the 'window' acts as a food and plaque trap and causes more damage than covering the gingival margin (Fig 5)(Lechner, 1985*b*).

To keep the gingival margin truly unaffected by the denture means a clearance of at least:

- 10 x 5 mm on the palatal mucosa in the maxillary arch (Fig 6).

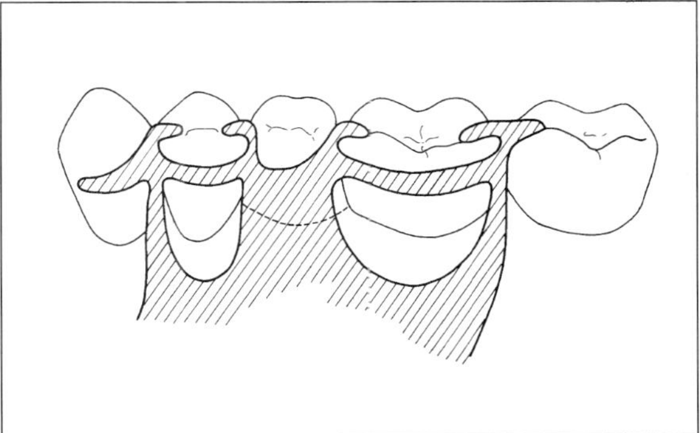

Fig **5** 'Small windows' on the palatal aspects of 24 and 26 act as food traps and cause more damage than covering the gingival margins. Such 'small windows' are to be avoided.

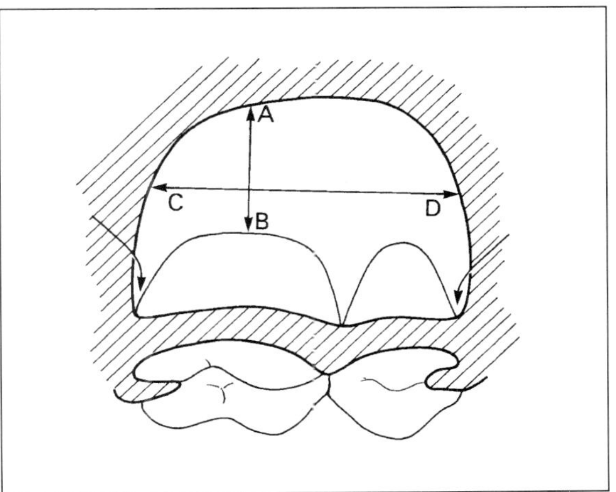

Fig **6** Maxilla. For gingival margin health, AB must be at least 5 mm and CD must be at least 10 mm.

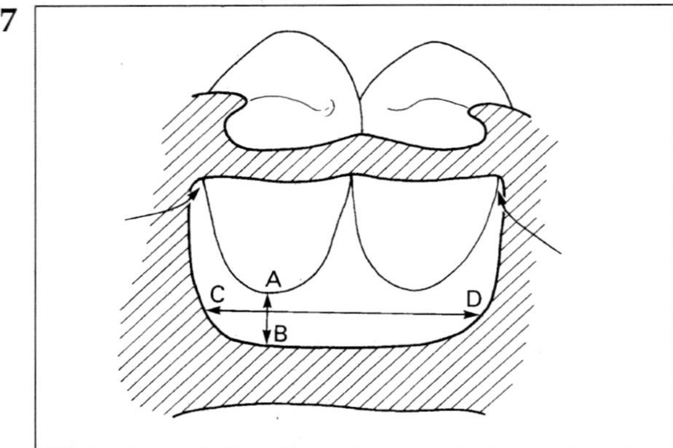

Fig 7 Mandible. For gingival margin health, AB must be at least 3 mm and CD must be at least 10 mm.

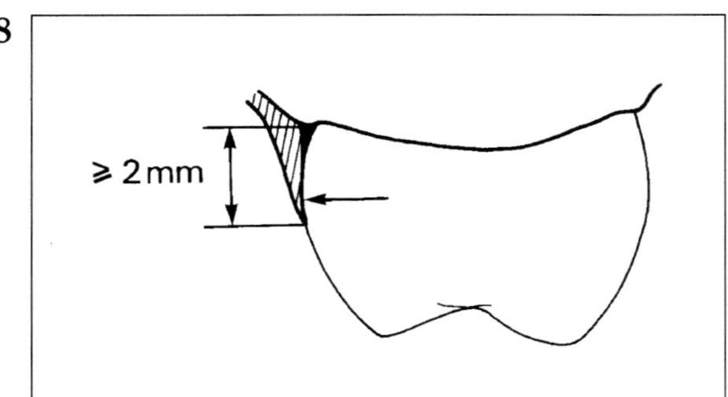

Fig 8 The palatal-lingual connector finishes above the survey line (horizontal arrow) and at least 2 mm above the gingival margin (the undercut is 'blocked out' between the survey line and the cervical region).

- 10 x 3 mm on the lingual mucosa of the mandibular arch (Fig 7).

Remember that food traps still remain where the denture base leaves the curve of the gingival margin (Figs **6**, **7**, arrowed), and the presence of the minor connector on the lingual or palatal surface of the abutments interferes with the streamlining of the denture.

- If you do need to cover the gingival margin, finish the denture on the tooth structure on or above the survey line and at least 2 mm above the gingival margin (Fig **8**).
- Keep clasps on the enamel and at least 1 mm clear of the mucosa and/or the cemento-enamel junction (Fig **9**).
- *Never finish any part of the denture on the gingival margin.*
- Keep denture components, for example direct retainers, to a minimum. Use indirect retention and guiding surfaces to make retentive units more efficient.

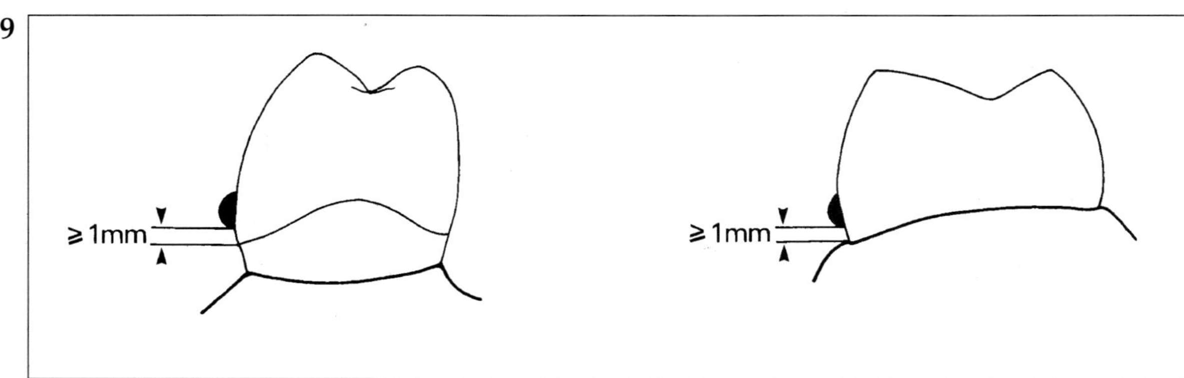

Fig 9 The clasp arm is on enamel and at least 1 mm clear of the cemento-enamel junction.

Occlusal integrity

If you intend to use the denture to change the patient's occlusal scheme:

- Any tooth modification must leave the occlusion *at least* as stable as it was before treatment began, while the patient is *not* wearing the denture.
- When wearing *either* the upper *or* the lower denture, the patient must be provided with a stable occlusion with maximum possible natural tooth contacts in the intercuspal position.
- When wearing *both* dentures, the patient must have a stable occlusion with maximum natural tooth contacts.

This also applies to *changes in vertical dimension*.

If you want to restore an overclosed vertical dimension you must do it so that the patient has a stable occlusion *without* dentures or with *one* or *both* dentures in the mouth.

If the vertical dimension is not overclosed, but you plan to open the vertical dimension because of overeruption of unopposed teeth and lack of space, then:

- Use the minimum amount of space consistent with adequate strength of the materials involved;
- Do not encroach on the speaking space;
- Keep within the limits of the free way space;
- Make sure that all the opposing teeth which have a natural occlusal stop are in contact with the denture at the new vertical dimension (Figs **10–12**).

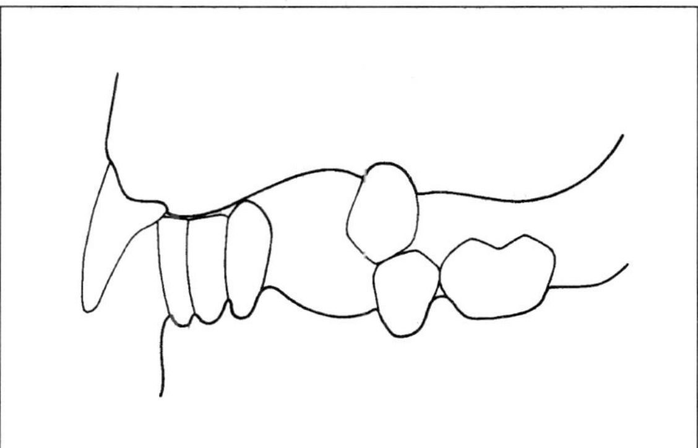

Fig **10** Lack of space behind the upper incisors necessitates a change in the vertical dimension of the occlusion.

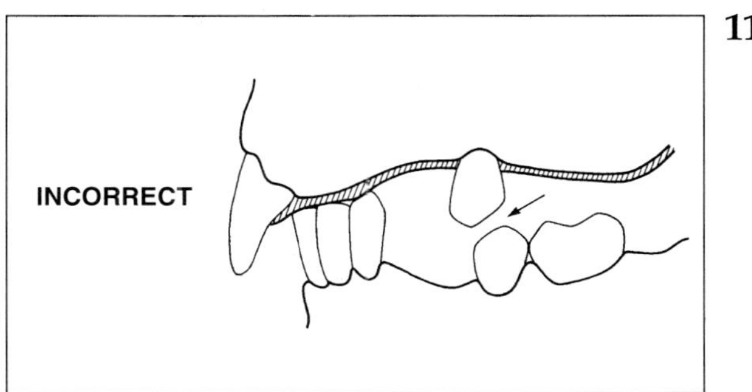

Fig **11** An increased vertical dimension due to the thickness of the denture behind 21 will feel uncomfortable as a result of lost contact between 24 and 35 (arrowed).

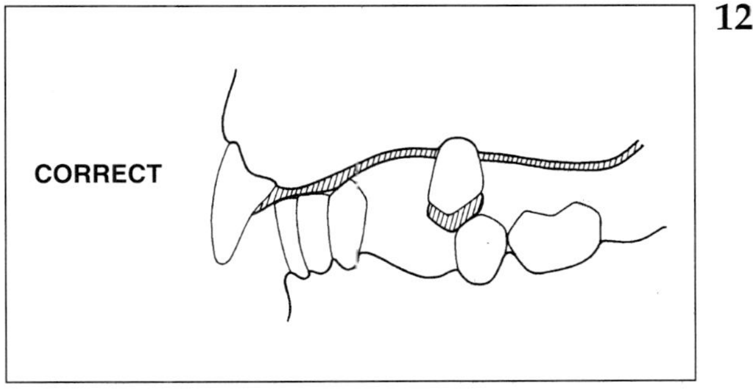

Fig **12** Increased vertical dimension due to the thickness if the denture behind 21 is equilibrated by the denture component maintaining contact between 24 and 35.

Oral hygiene and maintenance

Improvement and maintenance of oral hygiene is fundamental in all dental treatment. In RPD cases you will have seen the patient a number of times before deciding on the denture design and you are, therefore, in a very good position to know the hygiene standards set by the patient. Poor oral hygiene is exacerbated by any prosthesis in the mouth. Teach your patient how to look after his/her teeth and how to maintain gingival health.

In later stages, *recall and maintenance* are essential requirements for RPD success. Many RPDs fail because of lack of patient care and regular supervision by the dentist and hygienist.

An RPD which no longer fits will increase the torque on the abutment teeth as the dentures move in all directions on the tissues. Dentures with DEBs which no longer fit as the ridge resorbs are also prone to become sore at their distal extremity as they move on the oral tissues (Fig **13**).

Relining ill-fitting DEBs and *readjusting* the occlusion will make them more comfortable and will lessen the potentially traumatic torquing forces on the abutment teeth.

Resistance to various forces

The mechanics of denture design relate to providing resistance to the various forces that can be expected to act on it, and these are outlined in Chapter 3.

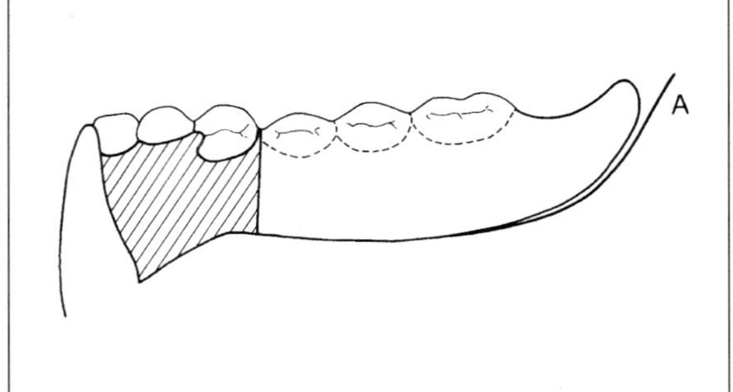

Fig **13** Point A is likely to become painful in function. Simply cutting back the denture in the region of the sore spot will not help. In fact, it will usually aggravate the problem by allowing more movement to occur.

3 Design Procedures: Resistance to Various Forces

With these design principles in mind, use the following checklist to design your denture. Use a sharp HB pencil to draw the design on to the surveyed study casts as you go. The drawing will indicate the precise positions of denture components in relation to anatomic features of the particular case. You should also draw the design on a prescription card (laboratory sheet) in ink (pages 55–56).

The drawing on the laboratory sheet is a plan view or two-dimensional diagram of the design, and the outline on the cast is a three-dimensional design. Together they give clear directions which the technician can follow without any misinterpretation.

Checklist:

- description of base(s)
- support
- retention: direct (including reciprocation)
              indirect
              guide planes
- connectors
- stabilisation
- acrylic anchorage
- recapitulation and streamlining

Description of base(s)

Describe the bases as tooth supported or mucosa supported or a combination of both.

Bounded bases are usually tooth-supported and the outlines are limited to the restoration of lost tissue. DEBs are usually tooth and mucosa supported and must, therefore, cover as much area as possible.

Draw the outlines of the areas to be restored on to the cast.

Support

Support may be defined as the foundation on which a denture rests, and which resists displacement towards the tissues. It comprises the hard and soft tissues that bear the loads of mastication and clenching applied to the denture.

Support options in order of preferences are:

- Occlusal rests on premolars and molars.
- Cingulum rests on upper canines and incisors.
- Incisal rests on lower canines and incisors
- Tissue coverage in cases where edentulous areas require support from mucosa.

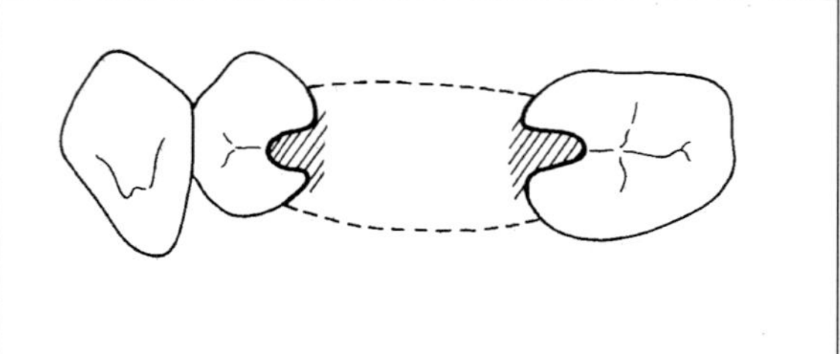

Fig 14 Occlusal rests at each end of a bounded base.

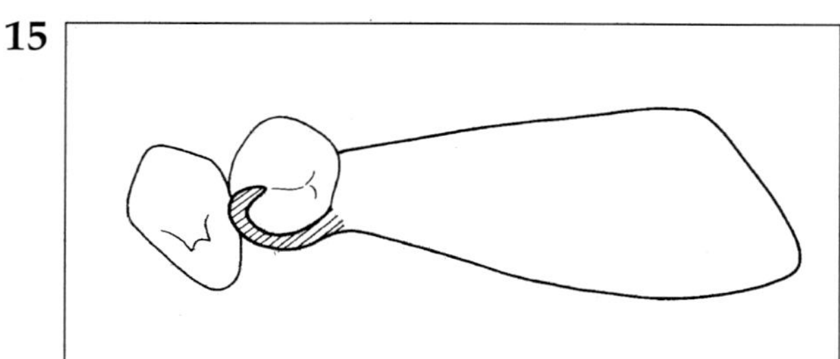

Fig **15** Occlusal rest on the mesial surface of an abutment for a DEB.

Occlusal rests

The most desirable vertical support is gained from occlusal rests which should be placed:

- Next to the edentulous area for bounded bases (Fig **14**).
- Away from the edentulous area for a DEB (Fig **15**).

ARE THERE ANY EXCEPTIONS TO THIS RULE?

The most important exception is related to occlusal integrity. *Never* place a rest where it interferes with a natural occlusal stop. Move the rest to the other side of the tooth (Fig **16**) or to an approximating tooth. If this is not possible, that is if all the teeth are in tight occlusal contact, try to find a specific area of tooth surface which will need minimum preparation for occlusal rest placement without interference (Fig **17**).

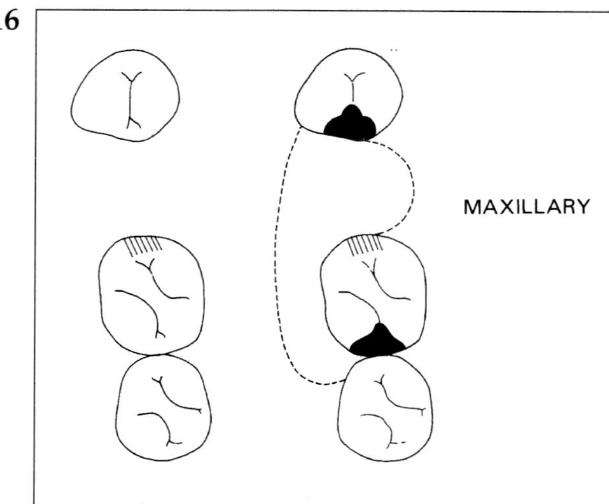

Fig 16 Occlusal contact on mesial marginal ridge of 26 (left); position the rest on the distal surface of 26 (right).

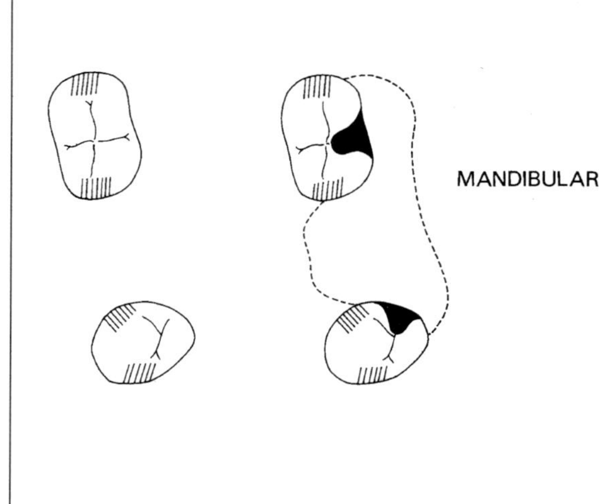

Fig **17** Occlusal contacts on the mesial and distobuccal surfaces of 45 and on the mesial and distal surfaces of 47 (left); position the rests on the distolingual surface of 45 and on the lingual surface of 47 (right).

Other exceptions to the above rules include:

- Bypassing a weak abutment and placing the rest on an approximating tooth (Fig **18**).
- Spreading the load by strategic placement of the rest on two abutments (Fig **19**).

Cingulum rests

Cingulum rests used for vertical support should be placed on upper canines and incisors.

Place a rest on the cingulum (or in the position of the cingulum where the anatomy is not distinct).

If there is occlusal contact with the opposing dentition on the cingulum, place the rest anywhere between this contact and 2 mm above the gingival margin (Fig **20**).

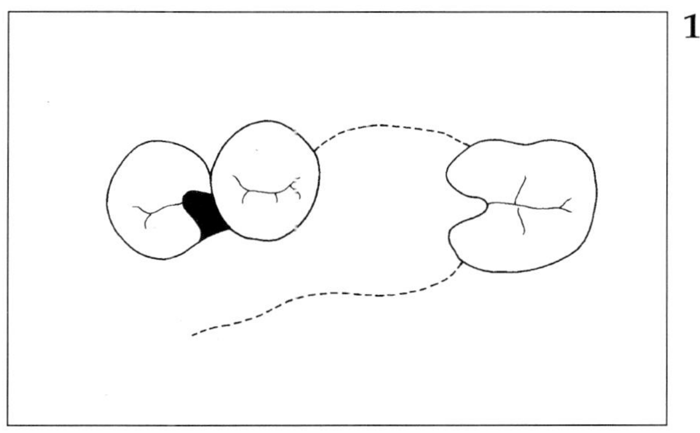

Fig **18** 45 has poor periodontal support. Position the rest on 44.

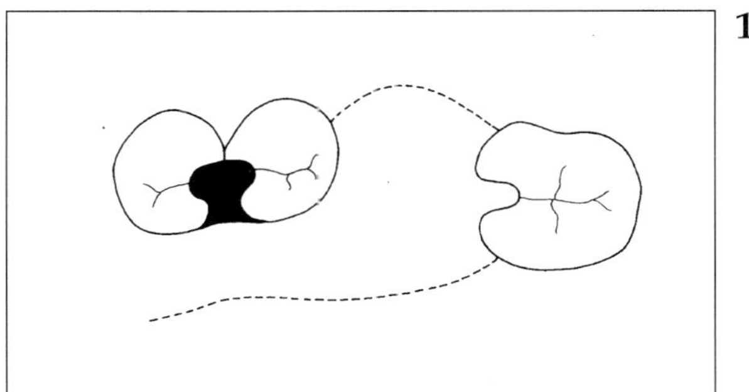

Fig **19** 44 and 45 are weak abutments. Spread the load between them by placing rests on both teeth.

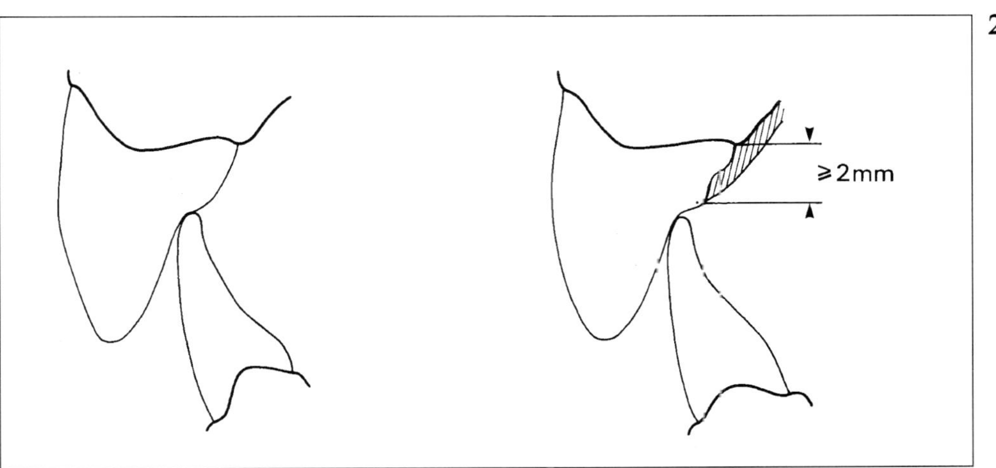

Fig **20** Occlusal contact between 33 and the cingulum of 23 (left); position the rest anywhere between this contact and 2 mm above the gingival margin (right).

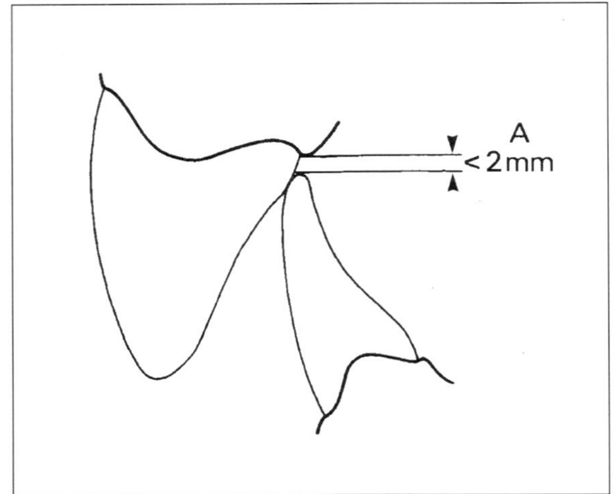

Fig **21** A is too small to allow a rest to be placed 2 mm above the gingival margin.

*What should you do if there is not enough space to do this as in Fig **21**?* In such a case:

- place the rest elsewhere, *or*
- allow the rest to act as an occlusal stop, but *remember* that using a rest to act as an occlusal stop cannot be done without a well-defined occlusal alteration plan (see Figs **10–12**).

Incisal rests

Incisal rests should be avoided wherever possible. They are unaesthetic and exert undesirable forces on the abutment teeth.

Where they cannot be avoided, incisal rests are used for vertical support on lower canines and incisors.

Never use an incisal rest on an upper incisor unless the incisal edge is broad labio-lingually and the rest seat can be prepared on the lingual edge.

On rare occasions, an incisal rest may be used on an upper canine if aesthetics and occlusion allow it, possibly in 'tooth surface loss' cases.

WHERE SHOULD INCISAL RESTS BE PLACED?
Incisal rests are often placed on two adjacent teeth to spread the load between them.

Modify the position of the rest for different circumstances as for occlusal rests (see Figs **16**, **17**).

Mucosal support

Mucosal support is used on edentulous areas which cannot be wholly tooth supported, that is DEB and very large bounded bases.

Bases needing mucosal support must cover as much tissue as possible, and usually have similar extensions as complete dentures.

Bases supported by *mucosa only*, that is without additional tooth support, tend to be more destructive and less efficient than those with other methods of support. Their use should be limited to some maxillary RPDs, or to very large mandibular DEBs.

Draw the support elements you have chosen on to the cast.

Retention

Retention is that property of a denture which resists outward displacement of the denture, away from the tissues.

- Remember that retention is not as important as *stability*.
- Try to *limit the number* of direct retainers to help preserve tissue integrity.
- Make sure each retentive unit works with *maximum efficiency*.
- Use your survey lines intelligently.
- Do not design rigid portions of retainer arms in undercuts.
- Remember that an active retainer arm should be reciprocated on the opposite side of the abutment.
- Improve retention by the use of *indirect retention*. Place direct retainers as close as possible to the edentulous area and indirect retainers as far away as possible.
- Improve the efficiency of retentive units with *guide planes* (also called guiding surfaces).

  RETENTION DEPENDS ON:

- Direct retention.
- Indirect retention.
- Guide planes.

Direct retention

Retentive pattern (strategic placement). Consider the stability of the retentive system and the fulcrum axis of rotation as in Fig **22**.

The best option is *three retainers* in a triangular arrangement set as far apart as possible. The third retainer prevents rotation about any pair of retainers and hence the retentive system is stable.

Use *more* retainers if:

- Available undercuts, or degree of undercut, are less than average.
- Guiding planes are short and/or few in number.

Use *two* retainers if:

- Only two abutment teeth are available, for example in a DEB. In that case indirect retention must be added as an extra component.
- Edentulous areas are small and undercuts and guide planes are optimal. In such cases, diagonally opposed retainers provide sufficient retention. The occlusal rests on the unclasped teeth will act as indirect retainers (Fig **23**).

Could *one* retainer be sufficient? One retainer is rarely used unless the edentulous areas are very small and the guide planes very long.

Decide what the retentive pattern will be.

Retentive units. Once the arrangement of the retentive pattern has been established, decide on the type of the direct retainers you will use.

Retainer selection depends on:

- The condition of the abutment.
- The amount of flexibility required.
- Efficient use of survey lines.
- The depth and magnitude of undercuts.

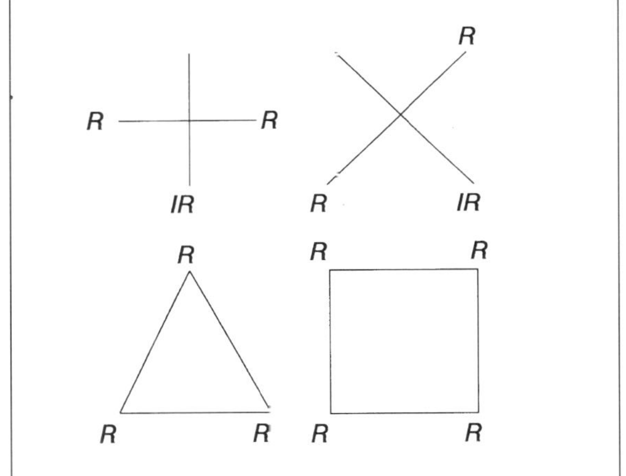

Fig **22** Retentive patterns R = retentive unit; IR = indirect retention. (After Taylor and Reese, 1984.)

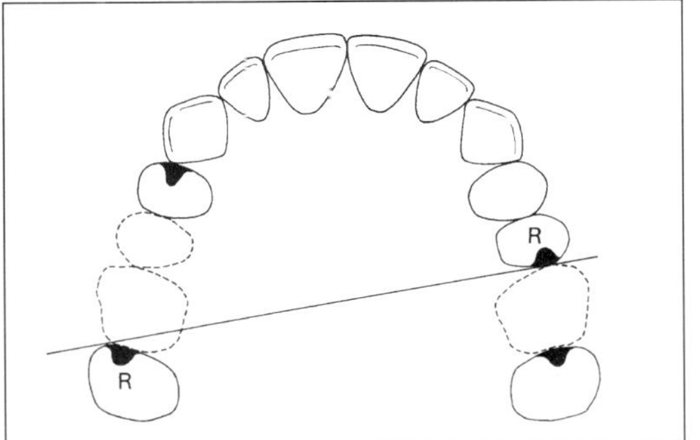

Fig **23** Direct retainers in optimal undercuts on 17 and 25 will provide retention if guide planes on all abutments are adequate. Occlusal rests on 14 and 27 provide indirect retention.

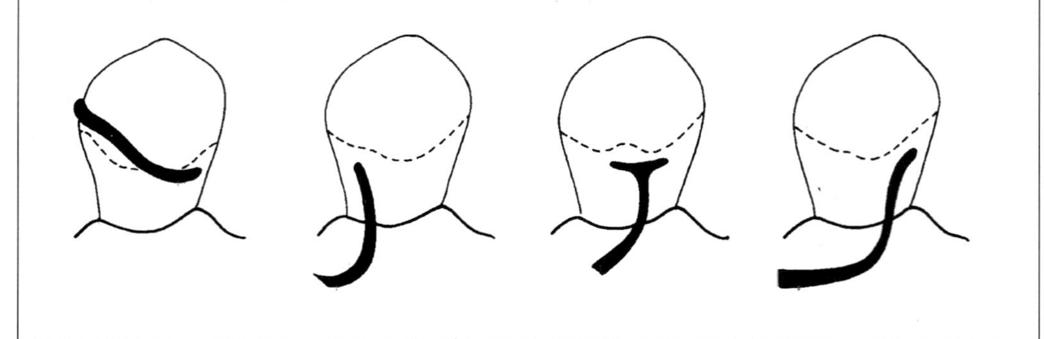

Fig **24** Various types of retainers have various degrees of flexibility – assuming they have the same cross-sectional area. More rigid (left) to more flexible (right).

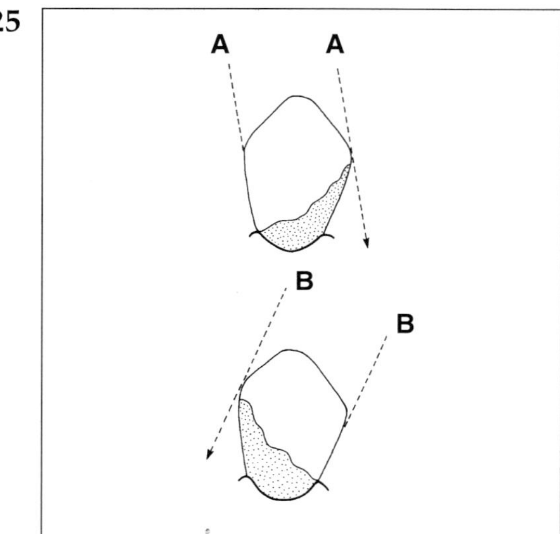

Fig **25** The path of insertion can be anywhere between A and B to give variations in the survey line and undercut position.

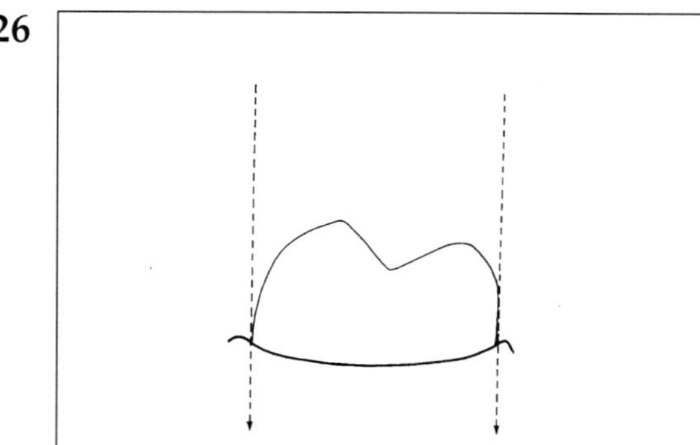

Fig **26** Tooth with no anatomic undercuts. Variation in the path of insertion will not produce a valid undercut.

- Soft tissue contour.
- Aesthetics.

CONDITION OF ABUTMENT

Whenever a tooth is lost, the tooth or teeth adjacent to the gap are affected by bone loss, which in turn depreciates the supporting periodontal membrane. This means that any additional load on an abutment in such a situation may have a detrimental effect. When placing a retainer on such a tooth is unavoidable, try to limit the loading by using a more flexible retainer.

AMOUNT OF FLEXIBILITY REQUIRED

The amount of flexibility required will determine the shape of the retainer and the material used in its construction (Fig **24**). Increased flexibility may be achieved by longer and/or thinner retainer arms. Remember, however, that the final mechanical properties of a retainer are decided by the level of technical expertise in the dental laboratory.

Materials in increasing order of flexibility:

- Cast cobalt-chromium.
- Wrought stainless steel.
- Cast gold alloy, correctly heat-treated.
- Wrought gold alloy.

EFFICIENT USE OF SURVEY LINES

Never design the rigid shoulder of a retainer to lie in an undercut area. The denture will bind in that area and insertion will be impossible unless the retainer is removed.

If you do not have undercuts in appropriate places, try changing the path of insertion and re-surveying the cast. You can change the size and position of undercuts (Fig **25**), but you cannot create undercuts on teeth which do not have them simply by tilting the cast (Fig **26**). If

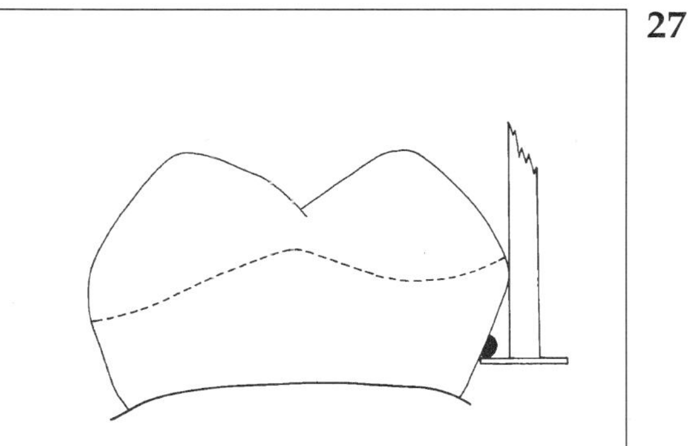

Figs **27**, **28** The depth of the horizontal undercut is indicated by the upper edge of the disc of the undercut gauge, which should coincide with the lower edge of the tip of the retaining arm.

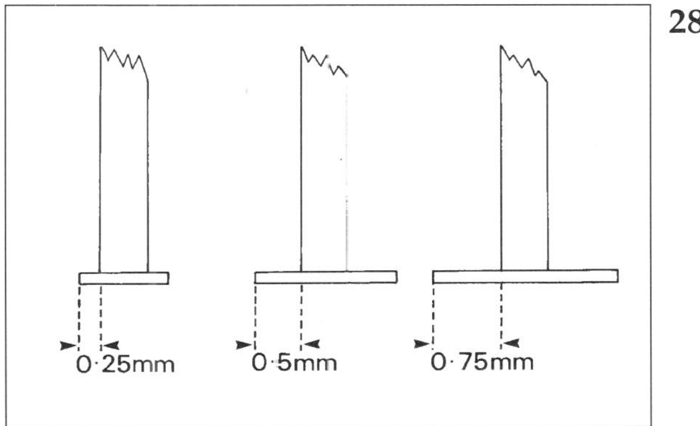

you want to create undercuts, you will have to modify the natural crown with a restorative material, for example, composite or gold alloy.

DEPTH AND MAGNITUDE OF UNDERCUTS

Undercut gauges allow you to measure the amount or degree of horizontal undercut present on a tooth surface and to locate exactly the ideal position for the retentive tip of the retainer (Figs **27**, **28**).

What size undercut should you use? For circumferential retainers, cast in cobalt-chromium, use a 0.25 mm undercut.

Vary this depending on:

- The retainer type (you can use a deeper undercut with a more flexible retainer).
- The material (you can use a deeper undercut with a more flexible material; that is, with low modulus of elasticity).
- The periodontal condition of the abutment (use a smaller undercut for a compromised tooth).

What should you do if the undercut is too large? Even if the horizontal undercut is very large, you do not need to use the greatest undercut area of the tooth surface. Decide what size undercut you want and place the retainer tip there (Fig **29**).

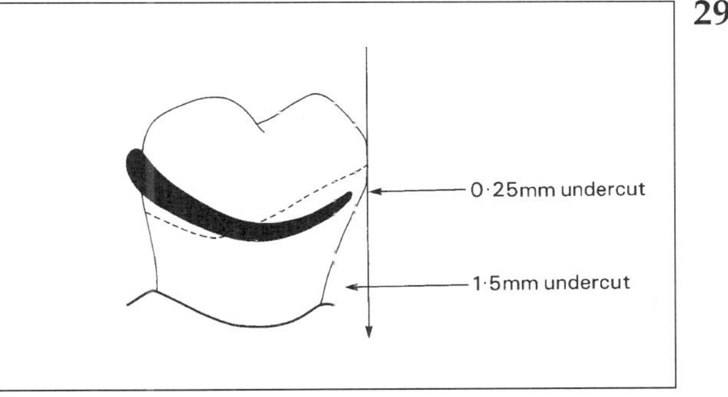

Fig **29** After deciding what undercut you want, place the retainer tip there.

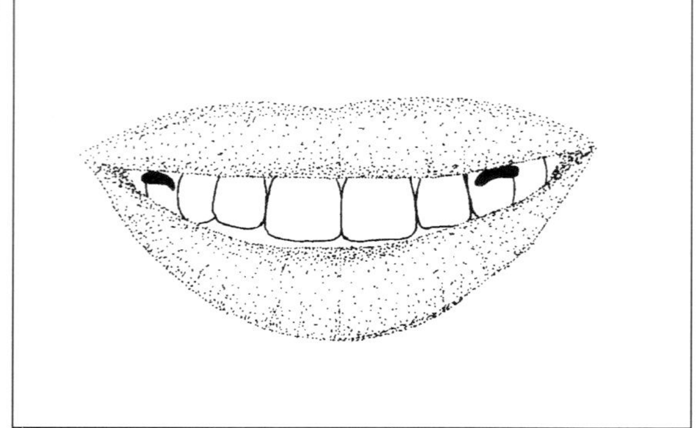

Fig **30** The retainer could spoil the patient's appearance.

What problems could this cause? This could cause problems with:

- *Aesthetics*. By having the retainer tip almost at the incisal or occlusal edge, the retainer could spoil the patient's appearance (Fig **30**).
- *Excess relief space* between the retainer arm and the surrounding tissues (Fig **31**).

In such cases, modify the tooth surface to lower the survey line and so reposition the desired undercut (Fig **32**).

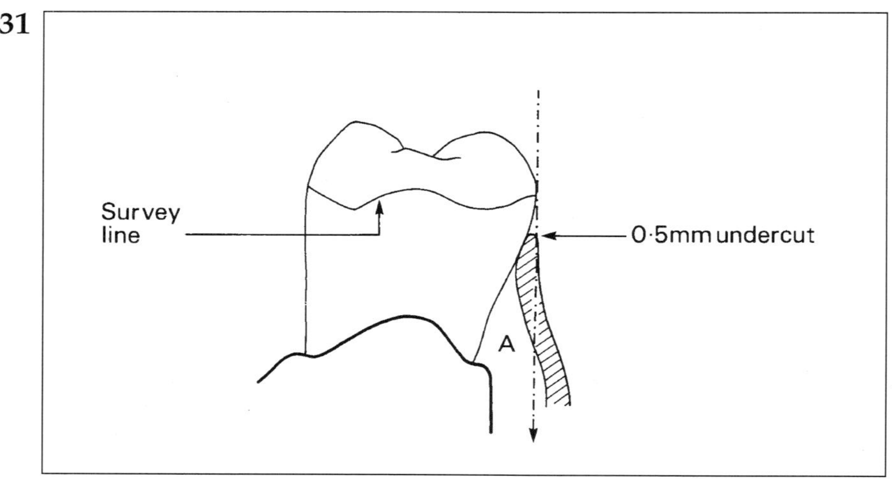

Fig **31** A large space (A) between the tooth and retainer arm could be a food trap. The arm could also cause irritation of the buccal tissue.

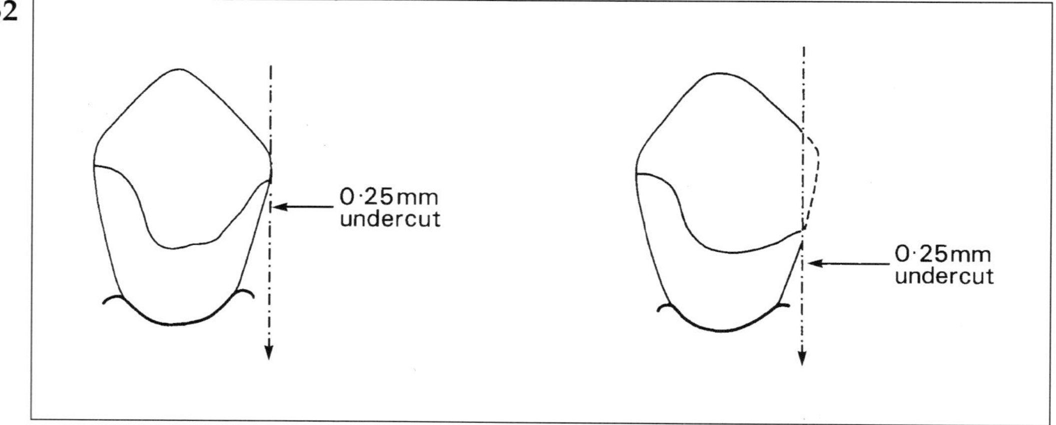

Fig **32** The tooth is modified to lower the survey line so that the retainer can still be placed in a 0.25 mm undercut, but closer to the gingival margin.

What happens if you put a retainer tip into too large a horizontal undercut? You will not be able to seat the denture in the mouth or, if you force it into place, you may not get the denture out.

But if you *do* manage to remove the denture you are likely to:

- distort the retainer arm beyond its proportional limit or
- break the retainer arm or
- damage the natural teeth or mucosa

What should you do if the tooth you want to clasp does not have a large enough undercut?

- Reposition the retainer on a different tooth.
- Use the smaller undercut with an extra retainer or retainers.
- Create a retentive area by making an inlay or crown or adding a microfine composite to the enamel surface.

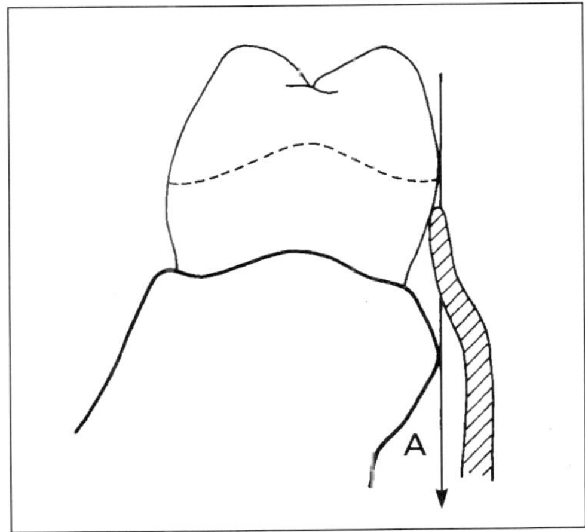

Fig 33 A large tissue undercut means a large space (A) between the tissues and retainer arm, which can harbour food and irritate the gingivae. The prominent retainer arm may rub against the cheek.

Soft tissue contour

Undesirable tissue contours may preclude the use of gingivally-approaching retainers. They may include:

- Excess tissue undercuts.
- Close frenal attachments.
- Unresorbed ridges.

Excess tissue undercuts. These will act in the same way as excess tooth undercuts in limiting the use of gingivally-approaching retainers (Fig 33).

Close frenal attachments. Frenal attachments may lie close to the gingival margins and, if broad and fan-shaped, may impede the correct location of retainers (Fig 34).

How can the two problems of tissue undercuts and close frenal attachments be overcome in cases where the design needs a gingivally-approaching retainer? Position the arm of the retainer in contact with the vertical slope of the acrylic flange. This will eliminate food traps and tissue irritation while allowing flexibility for the retainer to function (Fig 35).

In a design like this a tiny space must exist between the connector and the leading edge of the acrylic flange so that the retainer can flex. This space can be formed by 0.1 mm stainless steel tape, which can be withdrawn after the acrylic is polymerised. This tape leaves the acrylic with a polished surface.

Unresorbed ridges can cause problems with gingivally-approaching retainers where teeth are to be gum-fitted. The connector of the retainer can be bulky and ugly in such cases.

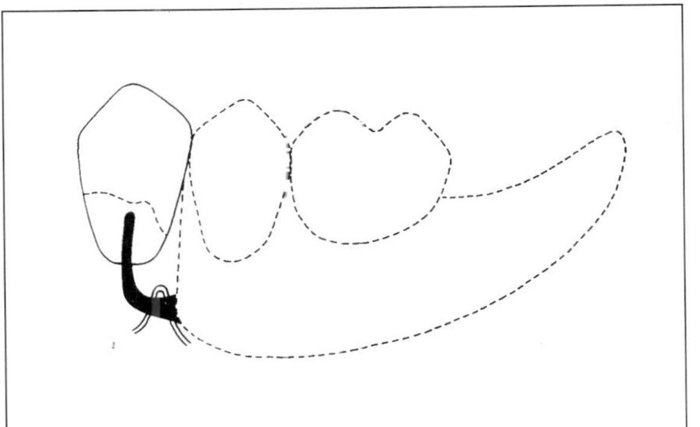

Fig 34 The arm of the gingivally-approaching retainer would cause irritation of the buccal frenum.

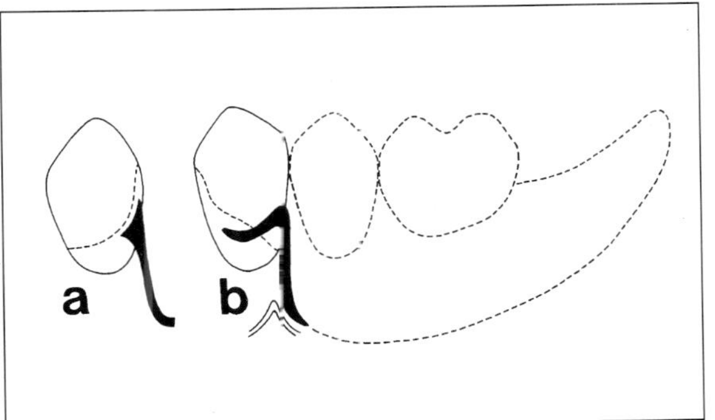

Fig 35 The retainer arm is in contact with the vertical slope of the acrylic, but it is free to move beside it (use either **a** or **b** depending on the survey line).

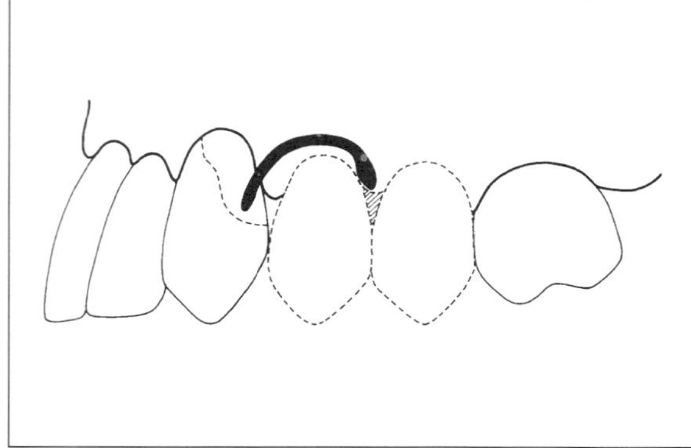

Fig **36** The retainer arm coincides with the interproximal space.

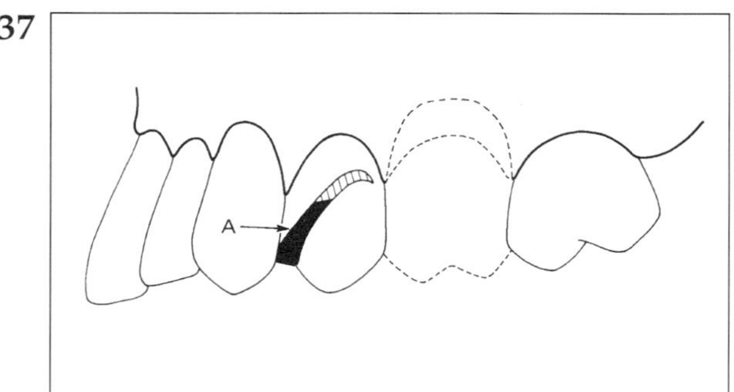

Fig **37** The bulky rigid portion (A) of the circumferential retainer is ugly on the mesial aspect of the premolar.

Try a different type of retainer. If this is not possible, position the minor connector of the retainer where it will coincide with an interproximal space (Fig **36**).

Positioning the minor connector in an interproximal space helps to reduce bulk, but will still be noticeable if the lip line is high.

AESTHETICS
'Ironmongery' in someone's mouth is seldom aesthetic. Try to minimise the amount of visible metal:

- Avoid circumferential retainers in the anterior part of the mouth.
- Keep the retainer tips as close to the gingival margin as is consistent with gingival health (ideally 1 mm above the cemento-enamel junction).
- Use distal undercuts with gingivally-approaching retainer arms where applicable.
- Use lingual or proximal undercuts for retention where applicable.
- Use extended guide planes where applicable.
- Relocate some retainers to less visible teeth.
- Omit some direct retainers and rely on indirect retention to gain stability.
- Avoid circumferential retainers in the distal undercut of premolars, that is, with the bulky shoulder of the retainer on the mesial aspect (Fig **37**).
- If you cannot avoid placing the retainer in a visible position, then sand-blast the alloy surface to reduce reflected glare and make it less obtrusive in the mouth.

Other aspects of aesthetics are discussed on pages 47–51.

Reciprocation

Check to make sure that all retainer tips are reciprocated by a rigid arm or by the denture base.

In deciding which method to use you should consider the health of the tissues and the streamlining of the RPD.

- A rigid arm will not be in contact with the gingivae but may cause a food trap.
- A denture base extension may damage the gingivae but will be more streamlined and possibly more comfortable.

Draw the direct retainers and reciprocators on to the cast.

Indirect retention

The term 'indirect retention' was coined to deal with the unique problems of DEBs. However, the concept of denture components functioning through lever action on opposite sides of a fulcrum is one which can be applied to all types of bases. For purposes of simplicity the term 'indirect retention' will apply to all such components in this text.

To use indirect retention:

- Locate the fulcrum line(s) indicated by the direct retainers.
- Find the perpendicular bisector.

The ideal indirect retainer is then an occlusal rest placed on this perpendicular bisector at a maximum distance from the fulcrum line (see Fig **38**).

When designing indirect retention remember that:

- It only works while the direct retainers function.
- It works best on the perpendicular bisector of the fulcrum line, which is the line drawn between the retaining tips of the direct retention units.
- It works better as the distance from the fulcrum line increases.
- It works best in an axial direction.

Such ideal placement is often not possible and you may need to rearrange your design and compromise with the type and position of indirect retention.

EXAMPLE 1 (MANDIBULAR DESIGN) (Fig **39**)
The 'ideal' indirect retention would transmit an axial force between 31 and 41 in the form of a well-defined cingulum rest.

This would not be possible without major restorative work due to the anatomic contours of lower incisors.

A *compromise* could be an incisal rest between 31 and 41. This would be very ugly and uncomfortable and is, therefore, unacceptable.

A *different compromise* could be a lingual plate resting on the (unprepared) cingulum of each lower incisor. This compromise sacrifices optimum support for optimal position. It can also be detrimental to gingival health.

Another compromise could be occlusal rests on the mesial aspects of 34 and 44, with extensions on to the (unprepared) cingulum of 33 and 43. This compromise sacrifices optimal position for improved support, that is, in an axial direction.

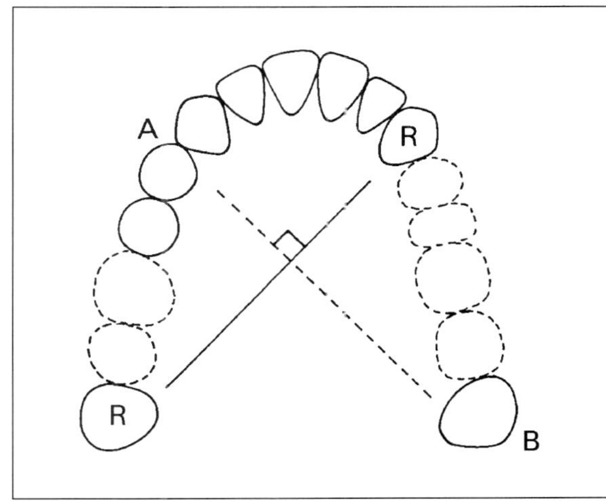

Fig **38** Ideal indirect retention is provided by occlusal rests at A and B (R = direct retainer).

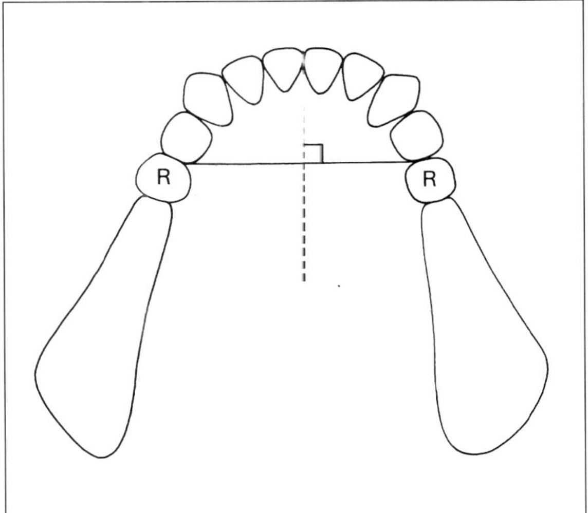

Fig **39** Mandibular design.

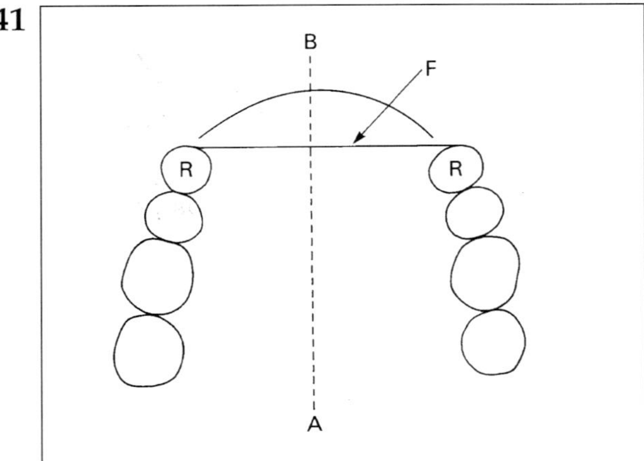

Figs **40, 41** The fulcrum (F) between the direct retainers (R) allows possible rotation towards points A and B.

EXAMPLE 2 (MAXILLARY DESIGN)(Figs **40, 41**)
'Ideal' indirect retention would be an occlusal rest at points A and B. This solution is obviously not possible.

To stop rotation towards point A: a *compromise* could be extension of the denture base over point A but this sacrifices optimal support, that is, mucosa support instead of tooth support, for optimal position.

Another compromise could be occlusal rests on the distal aspects of 17 and 27. This sacrifices optimal position for optimal support, that is, axially directed tooth support.

To stop rotation towards point B: indirect retention at point B is not possible. Therefore use *extra direct retention* at point A (use distal undercuts of 17 and 27) to prevent rotation towards B.

EXAMPLE 3 (MANDIBULAR DESIGN)(Fig **42**)
To stop rotation towards A: the *ideal indirect retention* would be an occlusal rest at A.

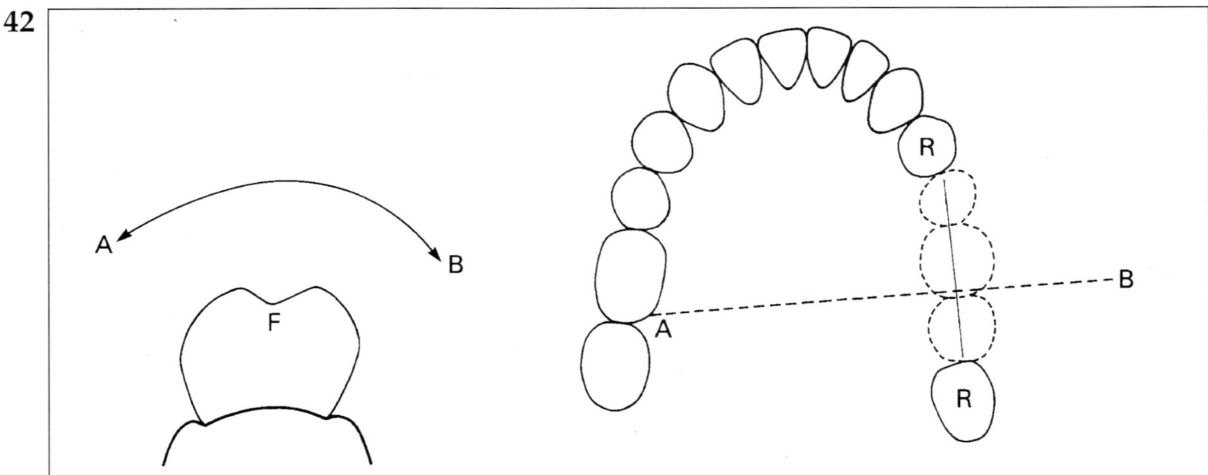

Fig **42** Direct retainers on 44 and 48.

To stop rotation towards B: add a *direct retainer* at A, giving a stable triangular retentive pattern (Fig **43**).

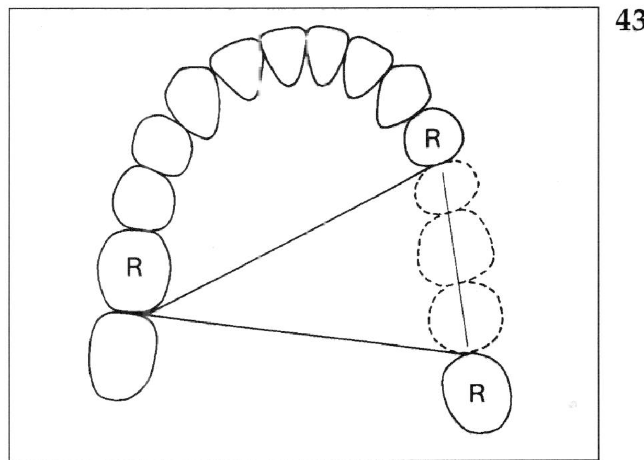

Fig **43** Triangular retentive system.

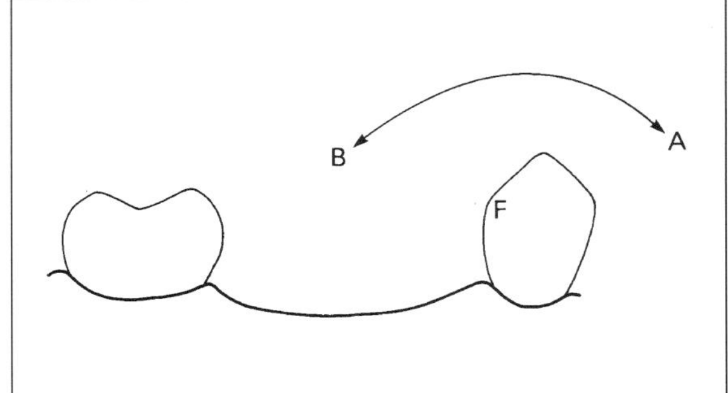

Figs **44–46** Mandibular design.

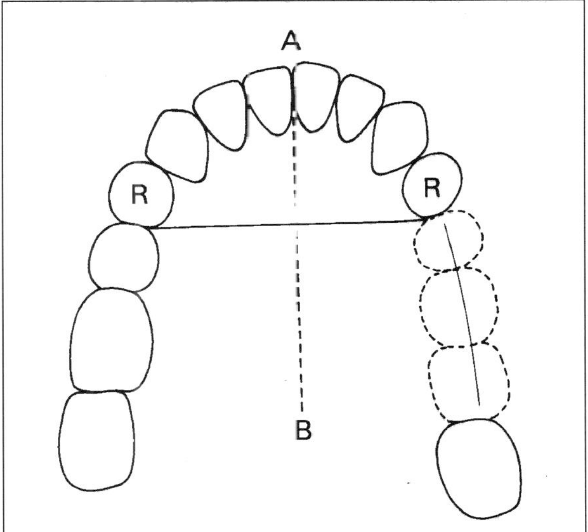

EXAMPLE 4 (MANDIBULAR DESIGN)(Figs **44–46**)
This is a different patient with the same teeth lost but with no undercuts on 48. This means that no direct retainer is possible on 48.

To stop rotation *towards A:* the ideal indirect retention would be on well-prepared cingulum rests on 31 and 41. This is normally impossible due to the anatomy of lower incisors.

To stop rotation *towards B:* no indirect retention is possible at B. *Compromise* by moving the fulcrum line. Place a direct retainer on 36 as shown below (Fig **46**). This changes the rotation points to X and Y.

Ideal indirect retention would now be at points X and Y.

Indirect retention can then be achieved easily at points C and D by placement of occlusal rests. The ideal position has been sacrificed for ideal support.

Check the design drawn on your cast to ensure that it has adequate indirect retention. Add extra indirect retention if necessary.

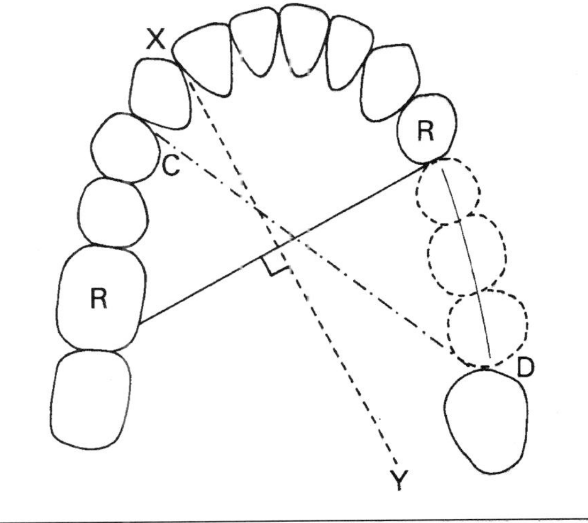

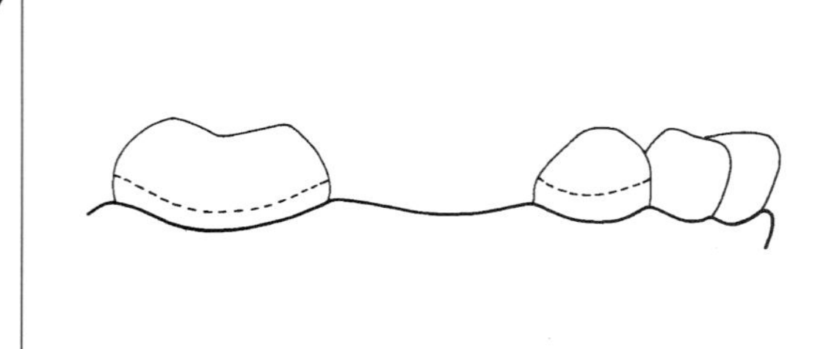

Fig **47** Very short guide planes will not help retention.

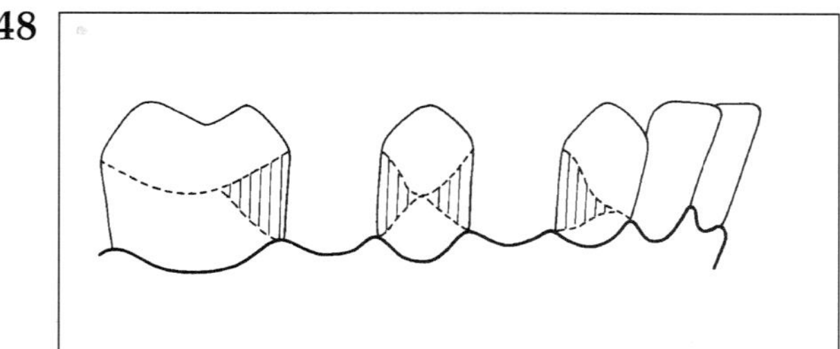

Fig **48** Long, numerous guide planes will markedly increase retention.

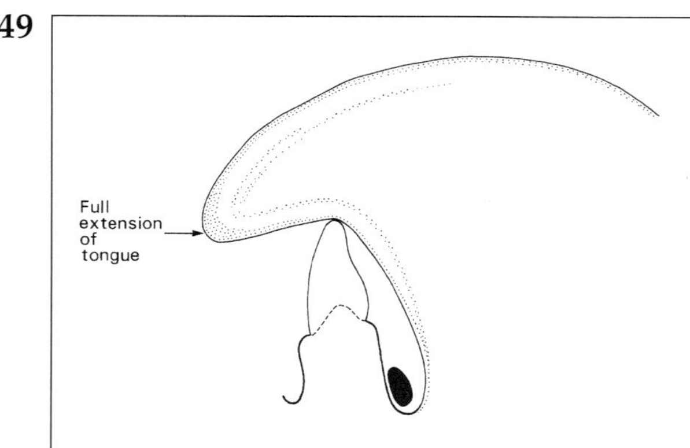

Fig **49** Placing of the lingual bar.

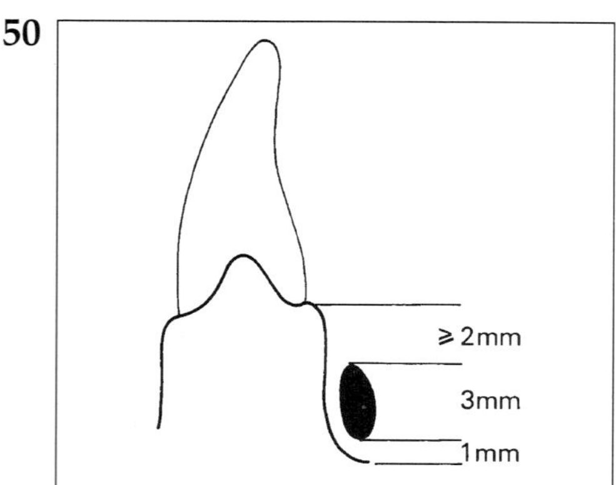

Fig **50** Minimum dimensions needed for the lingual bar.

Guide planes (guiding surfaces)

Guide planes increase the efficiency of direct retainers by:

- Defining the path of insertion and withdrawal precisely and thereby decreasing rotation.
- Frictional effects.

The efficiency of the guide planes will depend on:

- The number of guide planes.
- The length (height) of teeth involved (see Figs **47, 48**).

Use as many guide planes as possible to increase the efficiency of the direct retentive units. This usually means the judicious preparation of proximal surfaces of abutment teeth.

Draw small crosses on to the cast next to the tooth surfaces to be prepared as guide planes.

Connectors

All major connectors must be rigid. Make sure the dimensions of the connectors suit the material you are planning to use.

Mandibular connectors

There are various options and the final choice usually depends on the anatomy of the part. The options are:

- Lingual bar.
- Cingulum bar (dental bar).
- Lingual plate.
- Sublingual bar.
- Labial bar.

LINGUAL BAR

The most useful mandibular major connector is a lingual bar because it leaves the gingival margins uncovered. Use it wherever possible.

Where should a lingual bar be placed? A lingual bar should be placed at least 1 mm above the *correctly* muscle trimmed sulcus reflection (Fig **49**).

When can a lingual bar not *be used?* A lingual bar cannot be used:

- If there is less than 6 mm clearance between the lingual sulcus reflection and the gingival margins (Fig **50**).
- If the lingual tissues are excessively sloped (Figs **51, 52**).

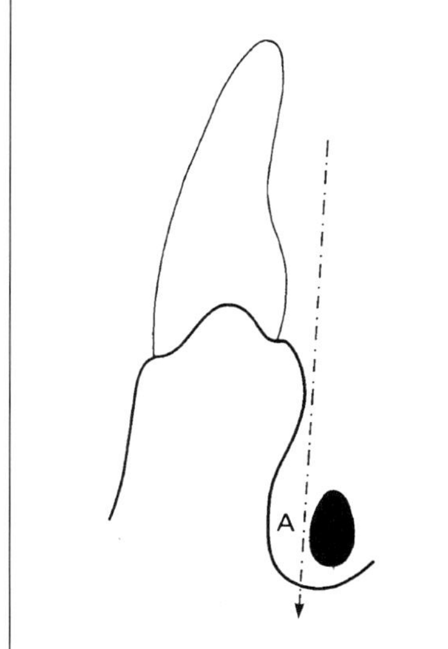

Fig **51** A large tissue undercut results in a large space (A) between the mucosa and lingual bar. This can cause discomfort and irritation of the tongue.

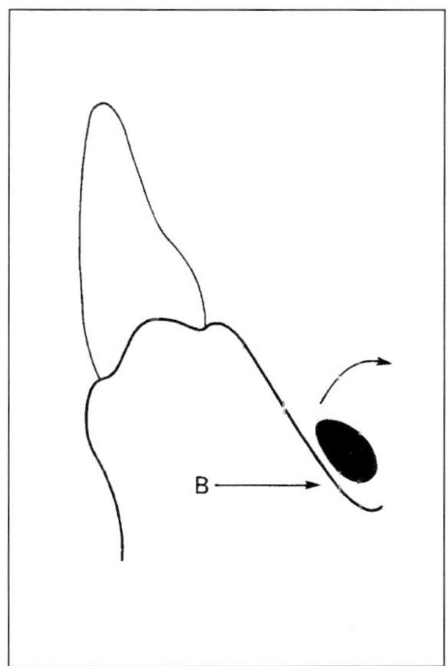

Fig **52** Tissue irritation is likely at B as the denture rotates in function.

Cingulum bar (Fig **53**)

Use a cingulum bar (dental bar) where:

- there is insufficient room for a lingual bar and
- the clinical crowns are long enough for the bar to be adequately rigid and
- there is good mesiodistal contact between the teeth

In certain cases where there is a well-defined cingulum on the lower incisors, or where you feel the cingulum bar has adequate tooth support, the lower edge of the bar can be made to fit against the curves of the lingual gingival margins. This method eliminates the space between the bar and the gingival margin which many patients find traps food and may exacerbate gingival trauma. Broadening the bar in this way also increases its transverse strength.

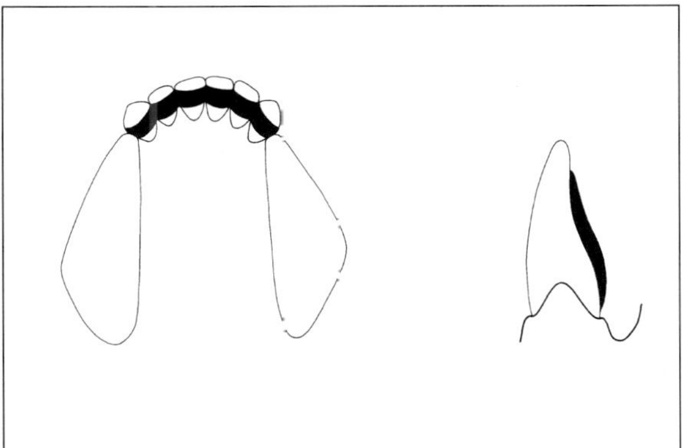

Fig **53** Cingulum bar.

Use a lingual plate if:

- A lingual bar is contra-indicated.
- A cingulum bar is contra-indicated.
- Indirect retention is needed and you feel that a lingual bar plus the necessary indirect retention component, for example, a Kennedy bar, would not be acceptable to the patient. The lingual plate provides indirect retention and is smoother and more comfortable, but it could compromise the covered gingival margins (Figs 54, 55).
- Do not use a lingual plate behind diastemata.

The outline form of lingual plates is restricted by anatomical limitations. Finish the lingual plate in the correctly trimmed lingual sulcus (Fig 56) or, if there is an undercut, at the height of contour of the lingual tissues (Fig 57).

The inferior part of a cobalt-chromium lingual plate is 0.7 mm, while the superior edge thins out to 0.35 mm to present a very thin covering around the incisor teeth. An acrylic plate has to be appreciably thicker and is, therefore, more likely to be uncomfortable.

54

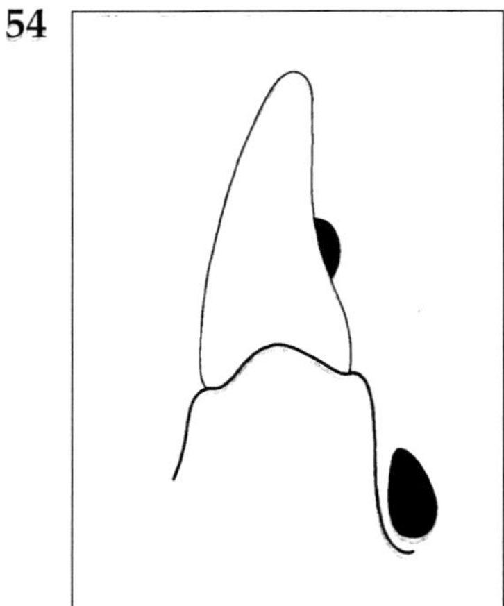

Fig **54** A lingual bar plus a Kennedy bar can be irritating to the tongue and unacceptable to some patients.

55

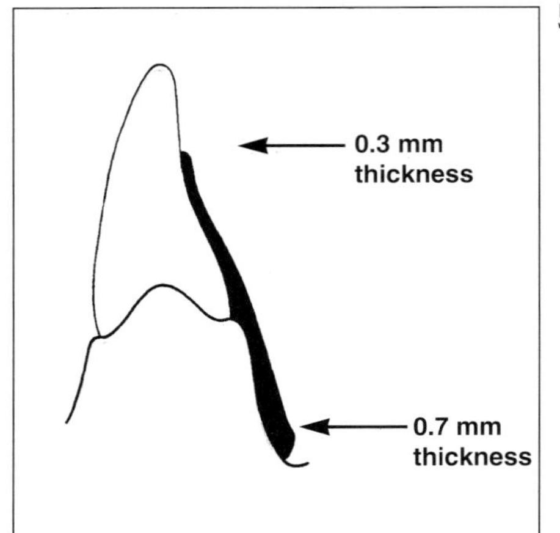

Fig **55** A lingual plate is smoother and more comfortable but compromises gingival margin health.

56

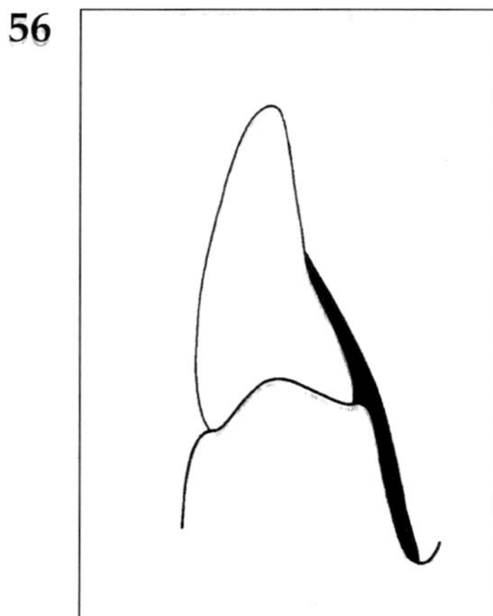

Fig **56** The lingual plate finishes in the correctly defined lingual sulcus.

57

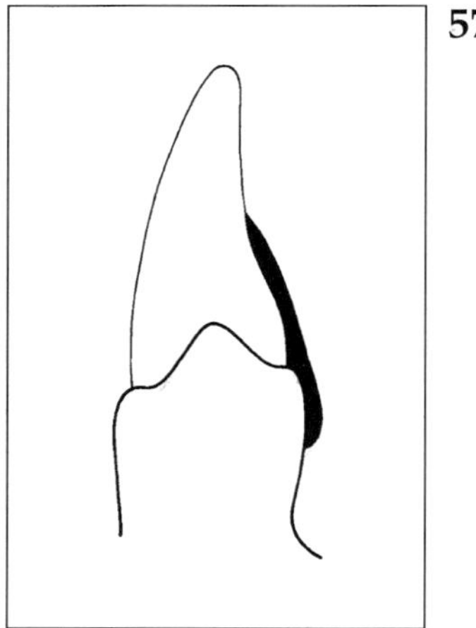

Fig **57** The lingual plate finishes at the height of contour of the lingual undercut.

Sᴜʙʟɪɴɢᴜᴀʟ ʙᴀʀ (Fig 58)
Use a sublingual bar where:

- There is insufficient room for a lingual bar.
- The patient has several diastemata.
- Specific indirect retention is not required. To position a sublingual bar correctly you need a very careful functional record of the sublingual area made in an accurate individual tray.

Lᴀʙɪᴀʟ ʙᴀʀ
Try to avoid this connector if possible. It is difficult to place and uncomfortable to wear, chiefly because it lies outside the anatomical alveolar contour and in contact with the lower lip, a very sensitive area. It is useful when the lower incisors are markedly retro-inclined or where there is a pronounced and non-negotiable torus mandibularis.

Draw the mandibular connector you have chosen on to the cast.

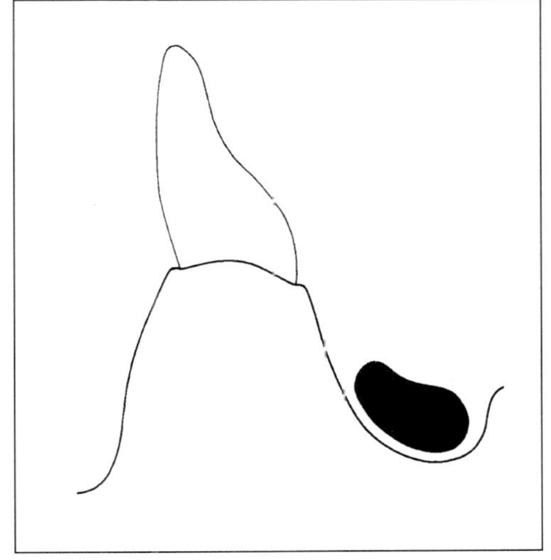

Fig **58** Sublingual bar. Note the kidney-shaped cross-section which gives the bar considerable transverse strength.

Maxillary connectors

Options:

- Mid-palatal bar.
- Posterior palatal bar.
- Anterior palatal bar.
- Ring bar.
- 'Horseshoe' plate.
- Full palatal plate.

Mɪᴅ-ᴘᴀʟᴀᴛᴀʟ ʙᴀʀ
This is the most comfortable maxillary major connector for the patient to wear. Vary the size and shape of the bar according to the shape of the palate (Figs **59, 60**).
    When should you *avoid* a mid-palatal bar?:

- Where there is a torus palati.
- Where the palate is very flat and hard.
- When edentulous area distribution makes it inconvenient; for example, multiple anterior edentulous areas.

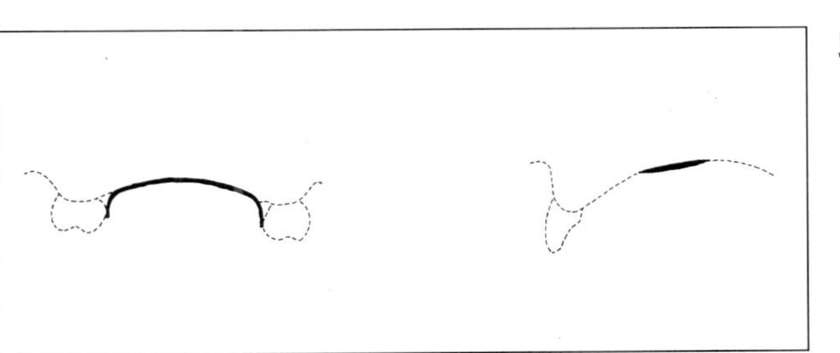

Fig **59** A flat palate needs a thinner and, therefore, wider bar.

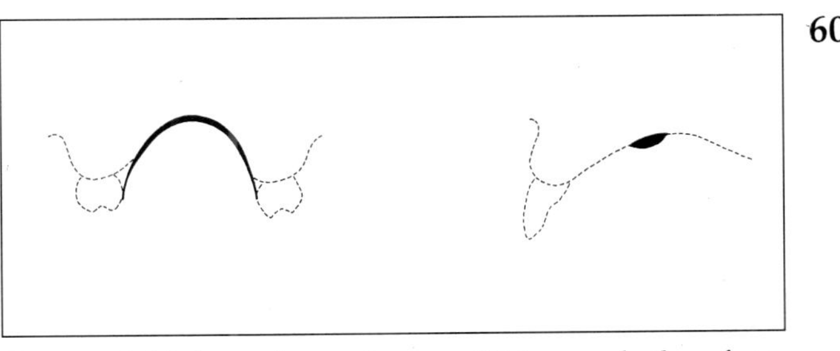

Fig **60** A high vault can have a thicker and, therefore, narrower bar.

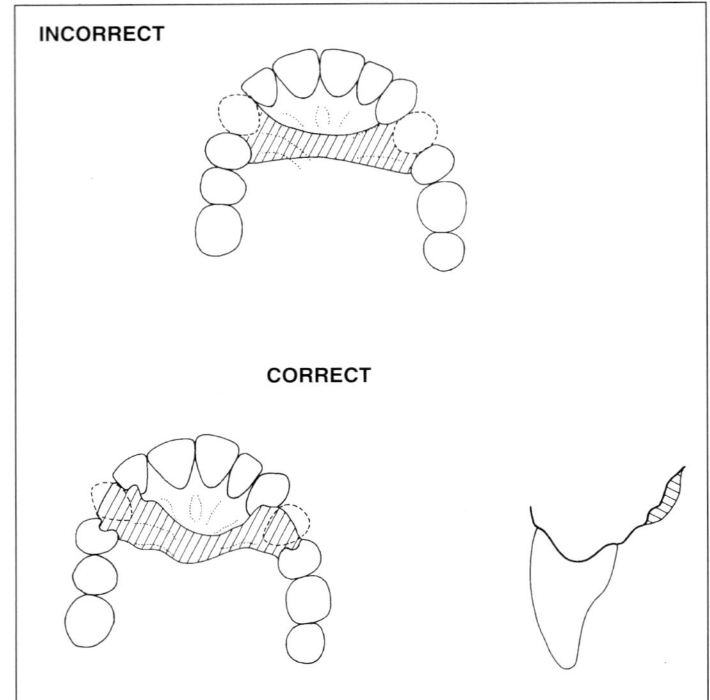

Fig **61** The palatal bar follows the contour of the rugae and tucks behind them to give a smoother, more comfortable finish.

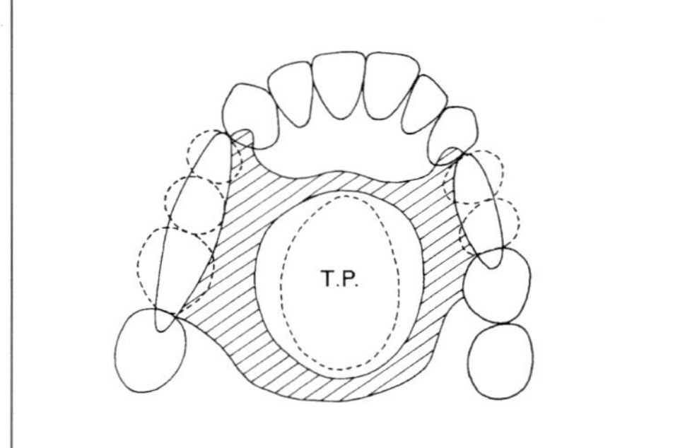

Fig **62** The torus palati (T.P.) precludes the use of a mid-palatal bar. A narrow anterior bar and a narrow posterior bar will give a strong 'ring' effect.

POSTERIOR PALATAL BAR

A posterior palatal bar is reasonably well tolerated by patients. Use this design where:

- A mid-palatal bar is contra-indicated.
- Edentulous area distribution makes it convenient.

ANTERIOR PALATAL BAR

An anterior palatal bar is usually not well tolerated by patients as it interferes with the rugae which are used as one of the main sounding boards during speech.

If saddle distribution is such that you need a bar covering the rugae, make sure it blends with the rugae and follows their contours, so that it is more difficult for the patient's tongue to detect the peripheral edge of the casting. Wherever possible, the edges of the connector should lie in the hollows between the rugae (Fig **61**).

RING BAR

A ring is a very rigid structure. A ring bar is, therefore, useful if the anatomical details of the case limit the size of a single bar and so make it flexible and weak. For example, in a case with a torus where there is very little space between the posterior extension of the torus and the fovea palati, a posterior palatal bar would be very narrow and, therefore, insufficiently rigid. Adding another, narrow, anterior bar will result in a strong, rigid 'ring' effect (Fig **62**).

'HORSESHOE' CONNECTOR

Use a horseshoe-shaped plate where there are multiple anterior edentulous areas. It is usually well tolerated by patients, but poor from a periodontal point of view, since it covers the gingival margins (Fig **63**). You may be able to keep some of the gingival margins uncovered as long as you remember the 5 x 10 mm rule (see page 11). Because of the broad outline of this design, a casting wax thickness of 0.5 mm will produce a cobalt-chromium base with sufficient transverse strength.

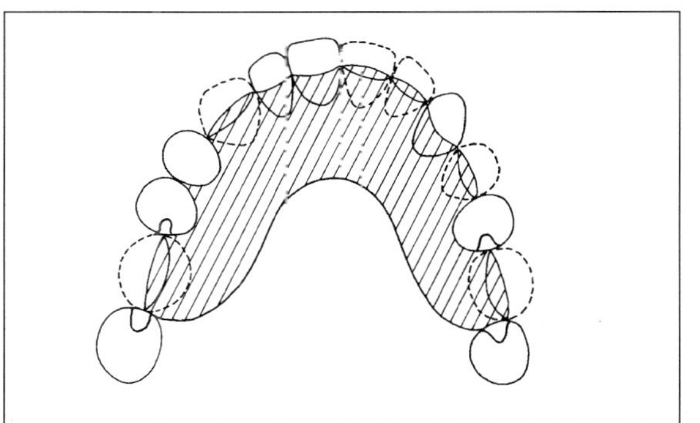

Fig **63** 'Horseshoe' plate.

FULL PALATAL PLATE

Use a palatal plate to provide maximum mucosal support. To do this it should cover as much of the hard palate as possible. Its posterior edge should lie in a position similar to a complete denture, that is, at the junction of the hard and soft palates.

Bringing the edge further forward usually makes the patient more aware of it as the edge is felt by the dorsum of the tongue (Fig **64**).

The thickness of a cast cobalt-chromium base should be 0.35 mm and all anatomical details, such as the lingual surfaces of teeth, gingival margins and rugae, reproduced. In contrast, an acrylic base would need to be thicker and without such detail.

Draw the maxillary connector you have chosen on to the cast.

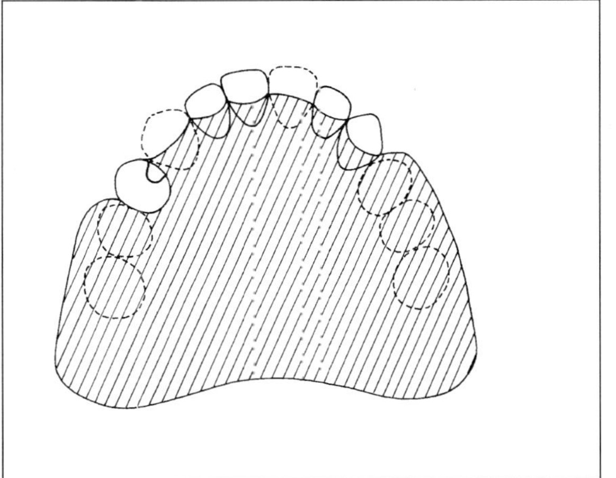

Fig **64** A palatal plate with maximum coverage.

Stabilisation

Stabilisation is that property of a denture which resists antero-posterior and lateral displacement.

Tooth-supported stabilisation includes reciprocators, guide planes and rigid shoulder sections of retainers. Occlusal rests can also offer lateral support if they have been specifically designed to do so, as are some types of prefabricated attachments.

With DEBs, remember to provide a component which will stop distal movement of the denture (see Chapter 4). Mucosa-supported stabilisation includes vertical sections of the ridge and/or palate (Fig **65**).

Check your design to make sure you have enough rigid sections to provide lateral and antero-posterior stabilisation. Modify the design where necessary.

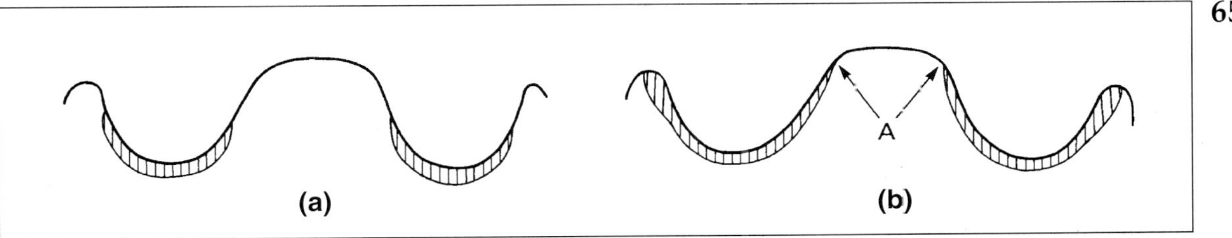

Fig **65** (a) Minimal lateral resistance. (b) The denture extends to the change of contour of the palate (A) giving good lateral bracing.

Acrylic anchorage and finishing lines

Map out the extension of the grids or mesh used for acrylic anchorage, the position of the finishing line and the placement of tissue stops.

Modify the acrylic anchorage where necessary for:

- Restricted interocclusal space.
- Additional anchorage.

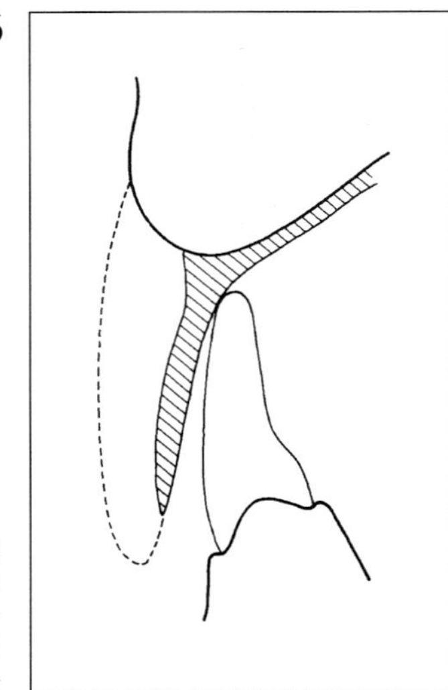

Fig **66** Metal backing providing strength where space is limited and anticipated occlusal forces heavy.

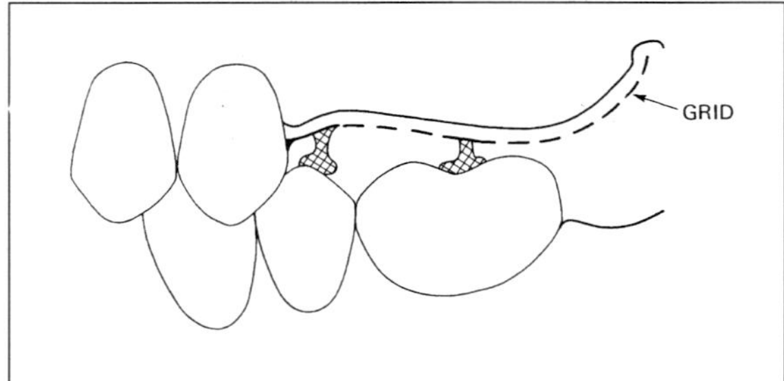

Fig **67** Metal stud extensions provide stable occlusal stops.

Restricted interocclusal space

- Use metal backing for anterior teeth where the opposing occlusion is very close and/or very 'heavy' (Fig **66**).
- Use metal studs extending from the grid to act as occlusal stops where posterior intermaxillary space is limited (Fig **67**). Denture teeth can then be simulated by forming tooth-coloured acrylic or light-cured composite around the stops.
- Change the position of the finishing lines to provide 'polished surface' occlusal contact where space is *very* small (Figs **68, 69**).

Additional anchorage

Use posts for:

- Isolated teeth.
- Gum-fitted teeth.
- All anterior teeth unless they are to be set in an adequate thickness of acrylic and/or the opposing occlusion is favourable.

Write any special instructions regarding acrylic anchorage on to the laboratory card.

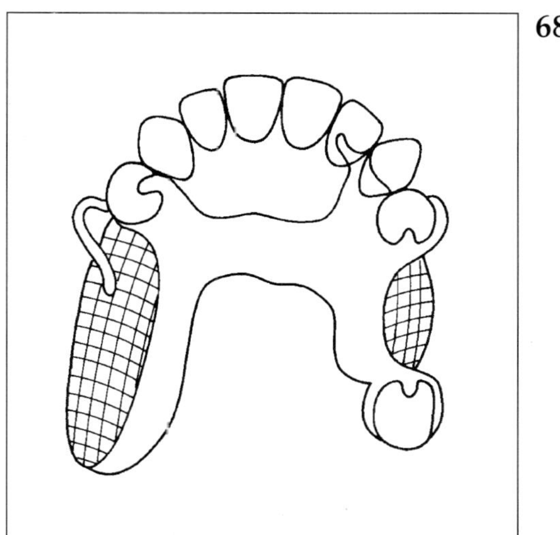

Fig **68** Usual position of the finishing line.

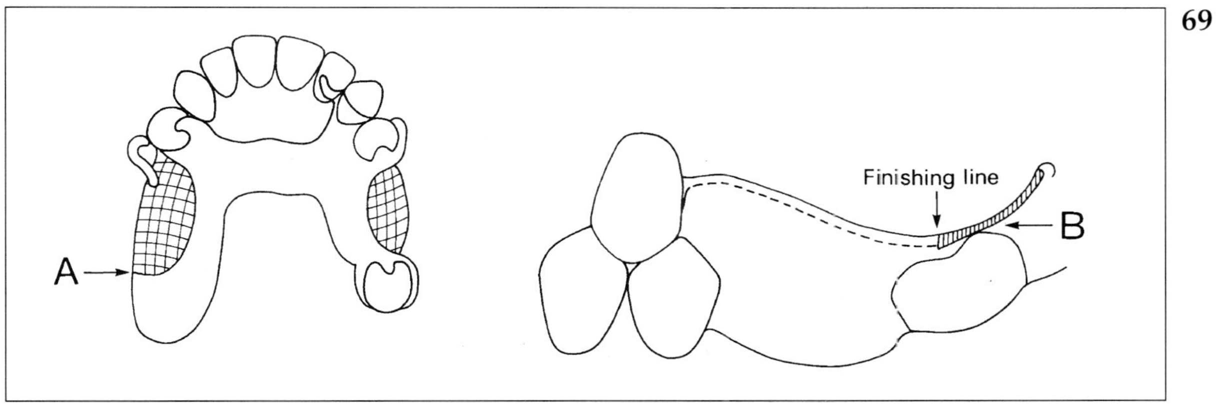

Fig **69** Modified position of the finishing line A to allow occlusal contact on the polished surface at point B.

Recapitulation

Check over the design as a whole and simplify it wherever possible. Add minor connectors where necessary.
    Check list:

- Everything must be connected.
- Have you avoided interfering with the occlusion?
- Have you considered the forces acting on the denture?
- Have you distributed the load equally?
- Have you avoided covering tissue unnecessarily?
- Have you avoided too many direct retainers by judicious use of guide plates and indirect retention?
- Is the design as aesthetic as possible?
- Are the components well supported and is the denture strong enough?
- Have you remembered streamlining?
- Will the denture(s) improve the mouth?

If so, complete the laboratory card and proceed through the stages of treatment.

4 Special Situations

DISTAL EXTENSION BASES

Removable partial dentures with DEBs are notably troublesome to make and to wear. They are very often unsatisfactory and, for that reason, extraction of distal abutment teeth should be avoided whenever possible. Even a remnant of an abutment tooth, such as the root of a hemi-sectioned molar after endodontic treatment, will serve as a useful abutment.

In many cases, you can omit a DEB from a partial denture design altogether, especially if it is unlikely to aid in the restoration of the occlusion. In such a situation, omission is better than inclusion in the overall design.

The problems presented by DEBs are twofold:

- Patients tend to find DEBs uncomfortable and unsatisfactory.
- The abutment tooth is more at risk than with tooth-bounded dentures.

Why do patients find DEBs troublesome? Patients tend to find DEBs troublesome because they lack the firm support which can be gained at either end of a tooth-bounded base (Fig **70**):

- When the patient puts pressure on the denture it will tend to 'bounce' due to the resilience of the mucosa.
- The patient will notice the difference between the feeling of pressure on the teeth (transmitted via the periodontal membrane) and pressure on the mucosa-supported denture.
- Direct retention is limited and indirect retention is often difficult, so that the denture tends to feel loose. Remember that movement of DEBs is not restricted to a vertical direction as usually depicted in drawings of DEBs. Equally important are sideways (bucco-lingual), and backwards (distal or antero-posterior) movements. This distal movement is a problem connected with the absence of a distal abutment tooth.

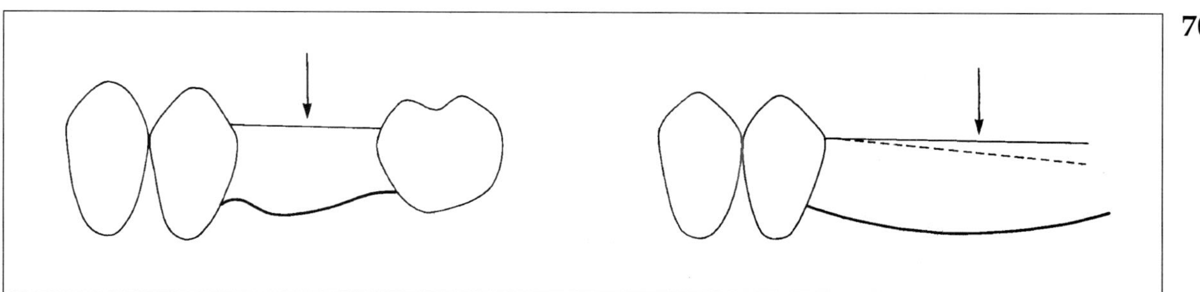

70

Fig **70** The tooth-bounded base has tooth support at each end (left); the DEB has tooth support at one end only. The other end can move on the more displaceable mucosa.

Why are the abutment teeth of DEBs at risk? The difference in compression of the periodontal membrane of the abutment tooth and the mucosa under the base means that all loads, even vertical ones, on the base are transmitted to the abutment tooth as torque (see Fig **71**).

Many laboratory and controlled clinical studies have been done regarding the resolution and final direction of these torquing forces. Taken overall, the results are inconclusive and no particular design

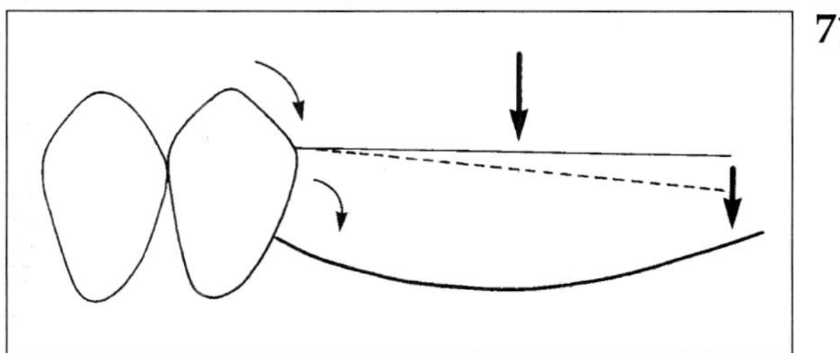

71

Fig **71** Vertical loads are transmitted to an abutment tooth as torque when the base moves in function.

philosophy has been definitively shown to be superior to the others.

However, longitudinal clinical surveys show that several factors can contribute to more comfortable and less traumatic DEB dentures (Anderson and Lammie, 1952; Koivumaa, 1957; Anderson and Bates, 1959; Lechner, 1985)).

What are these factors? In order of importance they are:

- Recall, maintenance and good oral hygiene.
- Mucosal support and stabilisation.
- Tooth support and stabilisation.

Recall, maintenance and good oral hygiene

Poor oral hygiene is exacerbated by any dental appliance and even the best-designed denture may cause problems. Teach your patients how to look after their teeth and gums.

DEBs which no longer fit will increase the torque on the abutment tooth as they move on the supporting mucosa.

DEBs which no longer fit as the ridge resorbs are also prone to become painful at their distal extremity as they move on the tissues (Fig **72**). Simply cutting back the denture will not help. In fact, it will usually aggravate the problem by allowing more movement to occur.

What should you do if the base does not fit? Relining ill-fitting DEBs and readjusting the occlusion will make them more comfortable and will lessen the potentially traumatic torquing forces on the abutment teeth.

Mucosal support and stabilisation

Mucosal support and stabilisation includes:

- Maximum tissue coverage.
- Functional impressions.
- Correct buccolingual tooth placement.
- Correct occlusal scheme.

MAXIMUM TISSUE COVERAGE
Because the base is largely mucosa supported, it is important to cover as much area as possible. This reduces the load per unit area.

What are the extensions of DEBs? The extensions of DEBs are the same as for complete dentures, and impressions for DEBs should be made in correctly extended custom trays so that the loose areolar tissues of the sulcus are not distorted.

In some maxillary DEBs, you may reduce palatal coverage where:

- There is good tooth support for the anterior section of the RPD.
- The opposing occlusion is light.
- The ridges are of good quality.
- The patient cannot tolerate palatal coverage.

Where the palate is not covered, the denture must extend into the hamular notches and the palatal finishing line should lie at the change of contour of the palatal tissues (Fig **73**).

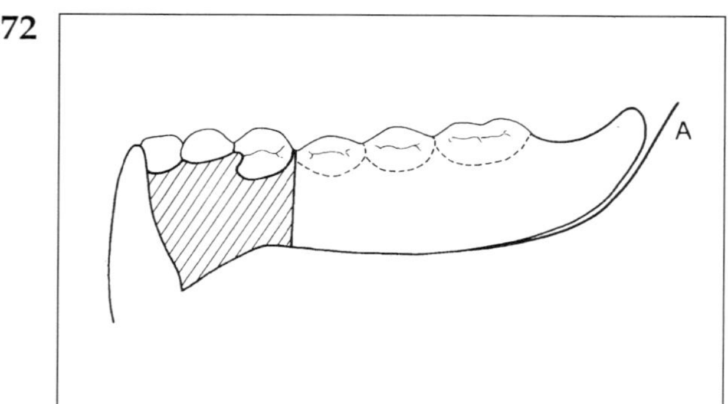

Fig **72** Point A is likely to become painful in function.

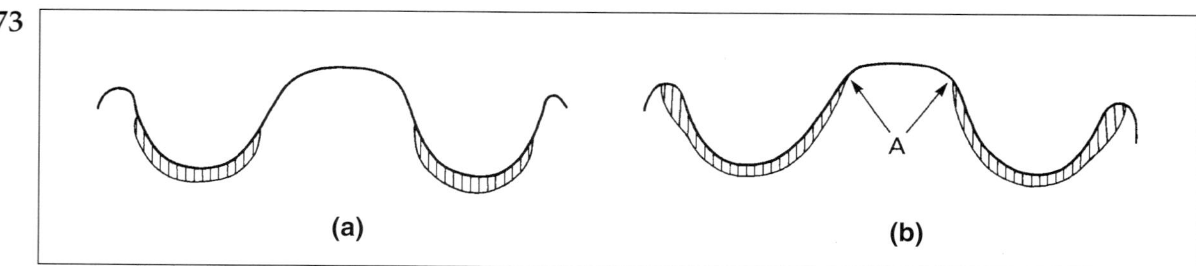

Fig **73** (a) Minimal lateral tissue support. (b) The denture extends to the change of the contour of the palate (A) giving good lateral tissue support.

Why are the extensions important? Although retention of an RPD is not altogether dependent on the periphery of the base being intimately related to the tissues of the sulcus, nor to the restoration of the sulcus anatomy, both are important in providing stability and support.

If the flanges are *underextended* in length or width, valuable support is lost and excess loads are put on the abutment tooth.

If the flanges are *overextended* in length or width:

- the peripheral tissues will be damaged as the muscles try to function, or
- the thrust of the muscles will overcome the retentive ability of the retainers and the denture will be dislodged.

FUNCTIONAL IMPRESSIONS

Functional impressions or tissue displacement techniques may occasionally be used to maximise mucosal support. The mucosa of the DEB area is compressed, so that the displacement of the mucosa relates to that of the periodontium when the denture is under masticatory or clenched load. Impression wax may be used in the altered cast technique, or the supporting tissues may be equilibrated by rebasing the finished denture, either at the time of delivery or after it has been worn for a few weeks.

CORRECT BUCCOLINGUAL TOOTH PLACEMENT

As with complete dentures, correct buccolingual tooth placement is important to allow the denture to lie passively in the neutral zone, so that the retainers do not need to retain against the forces of the cheeks or tongue.

Correct buccolingual tooth placement is more important than maximum intercuspation with the opposing occlusion. Consider the example in Fig **74.**

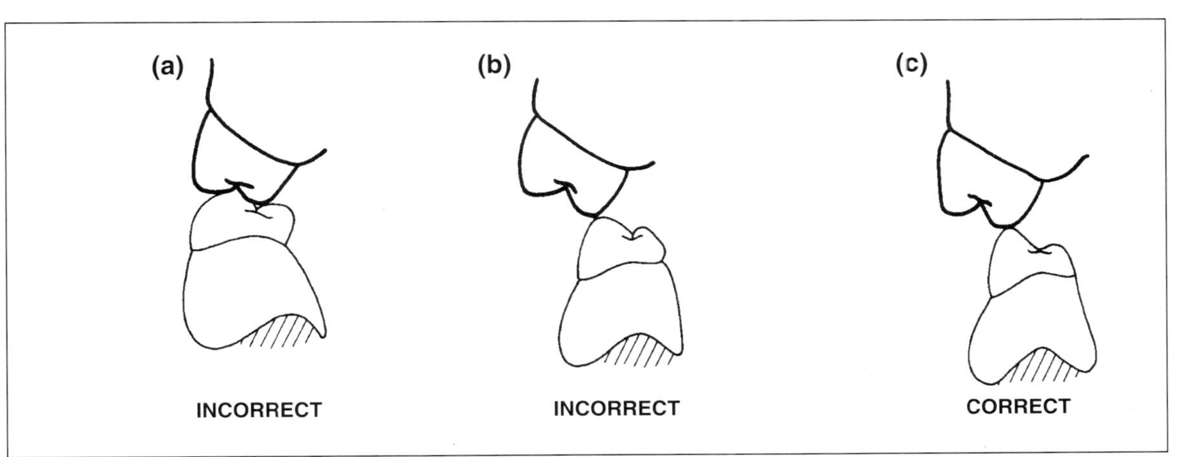

Fig **74** The maxillary natural molar has an exaggerated buccal tilt. (a) To gain maximum intercuspation, the mandibular denture tooth would need to be placed buccal to the denture-bearing area, thus causing instability of the mandibular denture. Such maximum intercuspation is contra-indicated. (b) Narrowing the width of the denture tooth and placing it in a correct buccolingual position may provide unstable point contact on the lingual incline of the lingual cusp of the maxillary molar, thus allowing further buccally-inclined eruption. (c) Minimal mouth preparation, flattening the maxillary lingual cusp tip and providing flat plane contact prevents overeruption and provides an occlusal stop.

Occlusal schemes relating to DEBs have the same two familiar aspects:

- Making the patient comfortable.
- Lessening the torque on the abutment teeth.

How can the occlusal scheme make the patient more comfortable? Clinical observation and clinical trials (Lechner 1985*a*) have shown overwhelmingly that patients are much more comfortable if they can achieve contact between their natural teeth, or between their natural teeth and the opposing denture if no opposing natural teeth exist (Fig 75).

Patients with dentures which preclude contact of natural teeth are likely to complain that:

'My mouth feels full of plastic'
'The denture is too big'
'I can't chew properly'

or similar phrases.

As in all RPDs, absolute precision in the occlusion of DEBs must be the aim of the clinician and technician. Modify the occlusal scheme to provide the maximum number of *natural* tooth contacts in the intercuspal position.

How can the occlusal scheme lessen the torque on the abutment tooth? To lessen the torque on the abutment tooth, you can:

- Keep the occlusal table narrow in the bucco-lingual direction.
- Shorten the functional occlusal table by keeping centric contacts close to the abutments. Remember that in the absence of symptoms, occlusal contact distal to the second premolar is only necessary to provide stability for a potentially unstable opposing denture, or to prevent overeruption of opposing natural teeth if no other option is available (see page 10).
- Ensure that there is no interference in eccentric movements. Provide balanced occlusion only in those cases where it is necessary for the stability of an opposing complete denture.

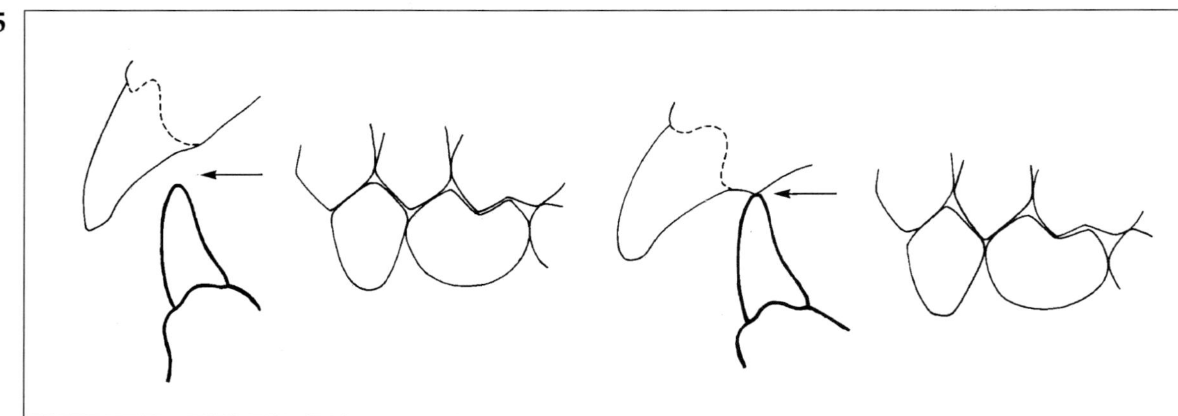

Fig **75** An occlusion propped open by a denture will feel bulky and uncomfortable (left); natural teeth contacting an opposing denture will feel more comfortable (right).

Tooth support and stabilisation

The survey line on the abutment of a DEB will only be valid if the tooth is encircled for more than 180°, that is, if some mesial component of the retention assembly prevents distal movement of the base (Fig **76**).

What kind of mesial component should you use? The best option is a mesially placed occlusal rest. This has the added advantage of directing torquing forces on the abutment in a mesial (favourable) direction.

If a mesially placed rest is inconvenient due to occlusal contacts, use a lingual or distal rest and a different mesial component, for example, a mesial guide plane (Fig **77**).

You could also use a *robust portion of a retentive unit* on a mesial surface or the *retentive tip of a retainer*. This is a poor option as the retentive tip is flexible and not designed as a stabilisation element (Fig **78**).

How can you further reduce torquing forces on the abutment tooth?:

- Use flexible retainers, the best option being a gingivally-approaching retainer, preferably wrought alloy.
- Avoid circumferential retainers.
- Augment the potentially poor direct retention by using indirect retention (see page 25);
- Consider using stress-breakers, but there are problems.

Stress-breakers are based on the belief that the action of certain parts can be separated from the movement of DEBs. Thus, when the term stress-breaker is used it is generally applied to a device that allows some movement between the mucosa-borne base and the rigid framework with its retainers and occlusal rests.

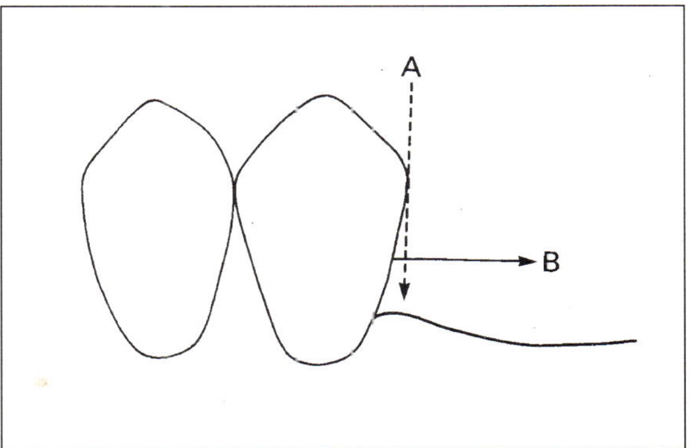

Fig **76** Surveying along path A without a mesial component in the retainer assembly will not be valid, because in the absence of a more distal abutment, the denture can dislodge along path B.

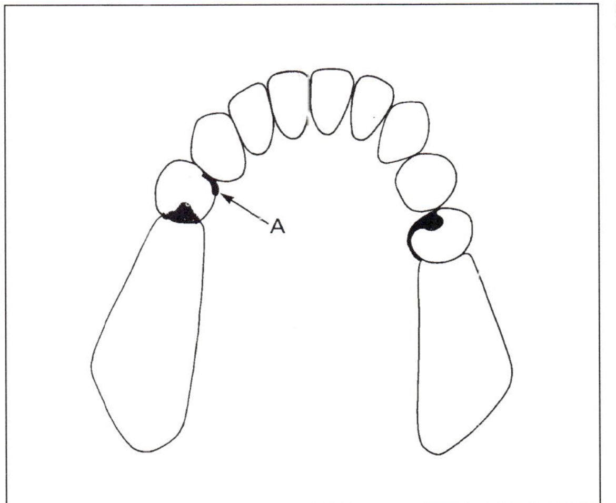

Fig **77** A prepared guide plane/plate on the mesial aspect of 34 prevents backward movement of the DEB.

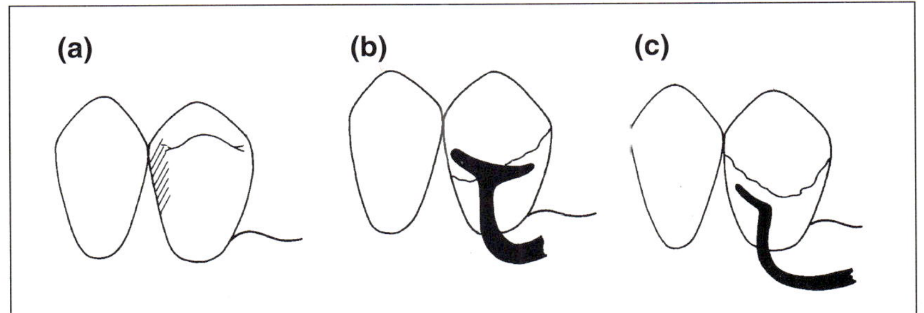

Fig **78** (a) Mesiolingual guide plane. (b) The robust portion of the T-bar (above the survey line) is on the mesial surface of the tooth while the flexible distal arm (in the undercut) gives retention. Note that the bulk of this clasp may be a contra-indication to its use. (c) Retainer in a mesial undercut.

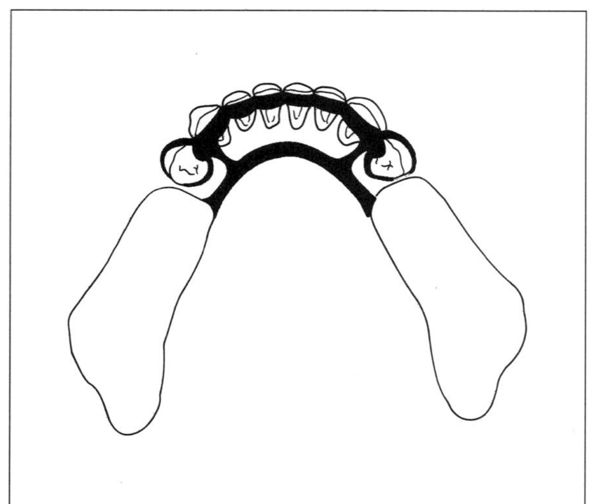

Fig **79** Cast lingual major connector with semi-flexible connectors.

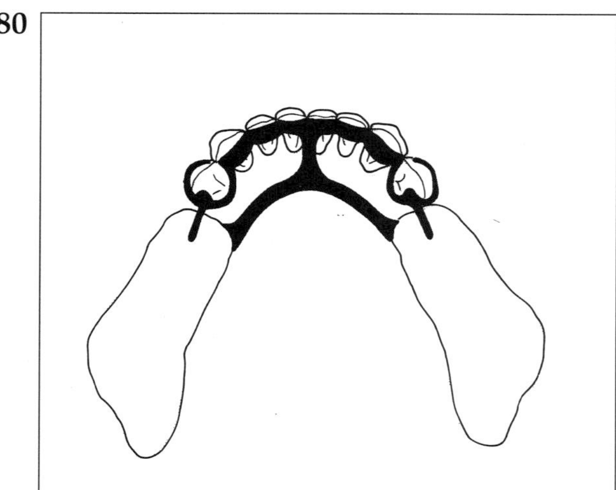

Fig **80** Mesial-facing clasps provide some indirect support for the free-end edentulous areas.

The aims of stress-breakers are:

- To direct occlusal forces in the long axes of the abutment teeth.
- To prevent harmful loads being applied to the remaining natural teeth.
- To share loads as evenly as possible between the natural teeth and base areas according to the ability of these different tissues to accept the loads.
- To ensure that the part of the load applied to the base area is distributed as evenly as possible over the whole mucosal surface.
- To provide greater comfort for the patient.

Many stress-broken designs are theoretically unsound. An example of this can be seen in Fig. **79**. This 'stress-broken' design does not function as expected because, when the edentulous areas are loaded, the denture rotates round the fulcrum axis through the occlusal rests. The distally-facing clasps do not prevent this rotation. Thus the denture behaves as if it was rigid.

Hinges are commonly used but they have the drawback of preventing an even load to the whole base area and, because of wear, causing an excessive lateral movement of the base.

Designs with stress-breakers need good retention in order to provide the necessary *indirect support*, because without retention the dentures behave in the same way as rigid designs. Indirect support means that the retainer on one side of a fulcrum axis through occlusal rests, can provide support for the part of the denture on the opposite side of the rests. For example, Fig **80** shows the mesial-facing clasps providing some indirect support for the free-end edentulous areas as the tooth-borne element tends to rise on load being applied to the denture. The fulcrum of rotation is through occlusal rests on the distal surfaces of the premolars. Distal to each retainer, and attached to it in the one-piece casting, is a vertical fin to resist lateral movement of the base. The anterior denture tooth is cut to fit over the fin, but with sufficient space to allow vertical movement of the base on the compressible mucosa. (For this reason, this denture tooth is sometimes known as the 'rider' tooth, analogous to horse riding.)

The continuous clasp (or dental bar) provides connection between the clasps and also indirect retention. The vertical fins provide lateral bracing for the bases, a particularly useful addition when the edentulous areas are long and the ridges are flat and atrophic.

In actual practice, however, it is seldom possible to make the clasping system sufficiently retentive to make the indirect support fully effective.

RPI design (Kratochvil, 1963; Krol, 1973)

Dentures designed with RPI clasping are rigid, but are intended to pivot around the abutment teeth without damaging the teeth or the mucosa. This design (Fig **81**) comprises an occlusal rest (placed mesially on the abutment tooth), a proximal plate (contacting a distal guiding surface) and a gingivally-approaching clasp (the I-bar), and is usually combined with functional impression techniques (see page 39).

The RPI system has two disadvantages. Because it is a 'system', it does not recognise any modifications which you may need to make for the individual needs of a patient. It also necessitates the use of a 'little window' on the lingual aspect of the abutment which could compromise gingival health (see pages 11–12).

Recapitulation

Avoid DEBs wherever possible. If they are unavoidable:

- Design the extensions and contours of the base as carefully as you would a complete denture.
- Place the denture teeth in the neutral zone.
- Adjust the occlusion precisely.
- Use light direct retention; place the emphasis on stability.
- Design the denture to counteract distal movement of the base.
- Provide for a good recall and maintenance scheme.

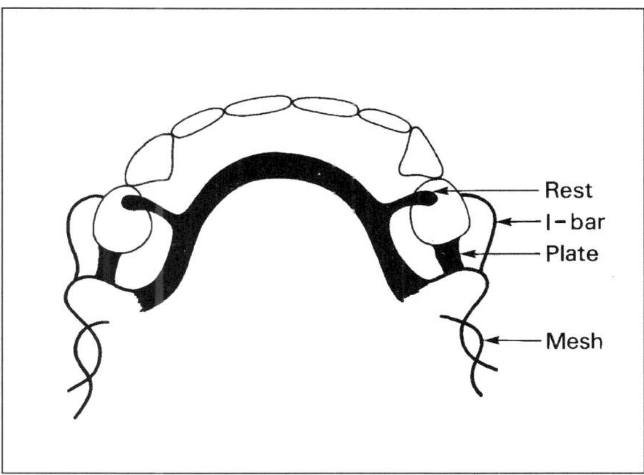

Fig **81** RPI design.

ANTERIOR MAXILLARY DENTURES

The problems of anterior maxillary dentures are:

- The magnitude and direction of the forces generated by the opposing occlusion (inward forces).
- The difficulty of finding suitable direct retention sites close to the base (outward forces).
- Indirect retention and the problems of rotation round a fulcrum.
- Aesthetics.

Occlusal forces

The natural dentition relies heavily on anterior guidance during function. When maxillary anterior teeth are lost, the potential for dislodging forces from the opposing occlusion is great (Fig **82**).

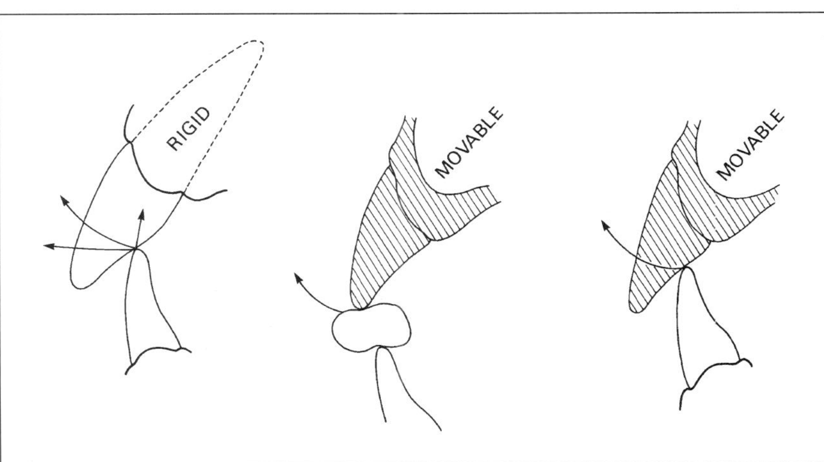

Fig **82** Natural dentition (left). Forces on artificial maxillary teeth tend to dislodge the denture in a forward and upward arc during incision of food (centre) and during empty movements (right).

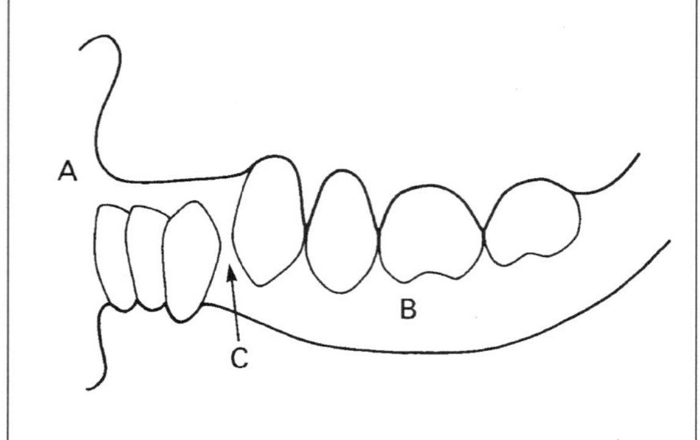

Fig 83 This case combines the problems of maximum rotational forces on the maxillary denture (A); a DEB opposing natural dentition (B); and no natural tooth contacts (C). It is one of the most difficult cases to treat.

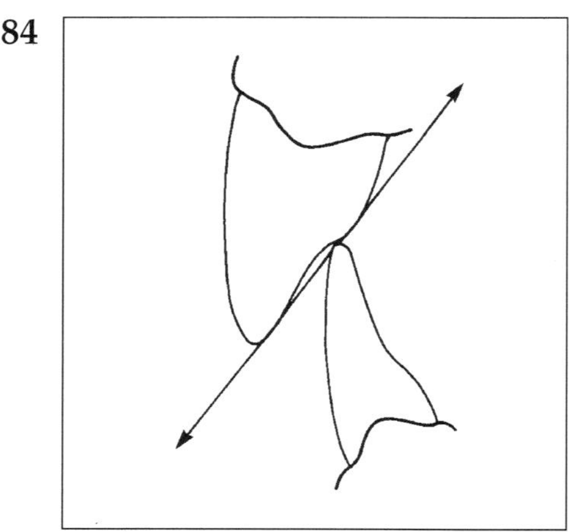

Fig 84 Steep incisal guidance in natural dentition provides anterior guidance during function.

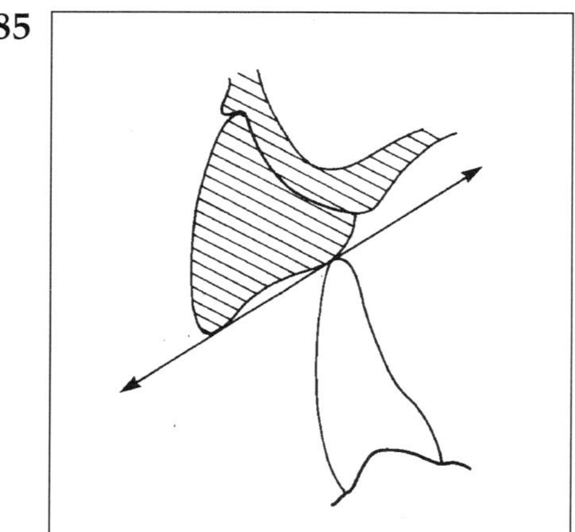

Fig 85 Artificial teeth shortened to flatten incisal guidance and allow group function or balanced occlusion.

These dislodging forces become more troublesome as more teeth are missing.

The *easiest* case is where only one maxillary incisor is missing. The occlusal load can be shared by the remaining dentition.

The *most difficult* case is where all six maxillary anterior teeth are missing. This is because there are no natural maxillary anterior teeth to take the load (anterior guidance). The difficulty here is greater if the mandibular incisors are present, and greater still if the mandibular posterior teeth are missing so that no natural occlusal stop exists (Fig 83).

How can you minimise these forces? Where the base is large you will have to consider establishing group function or balanced occlusion shared with the remaining dentition.

To achieve group function or balanced occlusion you may need to compromise aesthetics by shortening the upper anterior teeth to provide flatter incisal guidance (Figs 84, 85).

Is such a compromise to aesthetic tooth placement acceptable? Sometimes it is not acceptable. You have to consider each case individually. Weigh the importance of occlusal harmony against the requirements of aesthetic tooth placement, and reach the best compromise for the requirements of each patient individually.

Direct retention

Try to achieve direct retention as close to the base as possible, although this may be difficult to achieve due to aesthetic considerations and probable close occlusal contacts (Figs **86**, **87**).

The following are some methods of dealing with this problem.

Use an oblique path of insertion. Oblique means an upward and backward path of insertion which is different from the potential (downward) path of displacement. When in situ, the denture base itself acts as a retainer in the mesial undercut (Fig **88**).

The undercut at B has to be blocked out, and this creates an unfavourable zone of displacement of the posterior base. This necessitates the use of a retainer on the canine which, together with the acrylic in undercuts A and C, resists downward displacement of the denture at right angles to the occlusal plane.

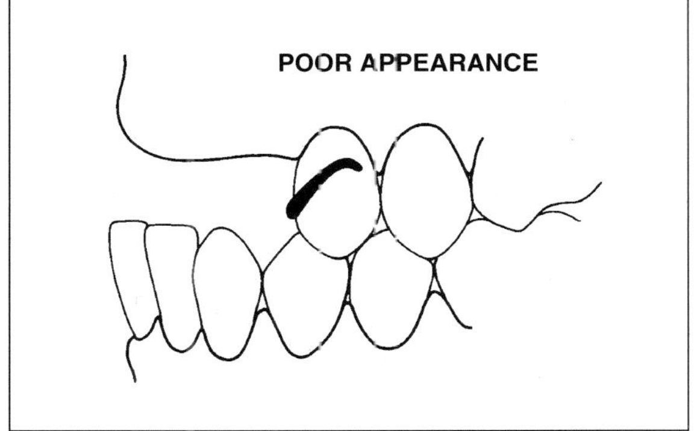

Fig **86** A circumferential retainer on 24 with a mesial approach would be unaesthetic.

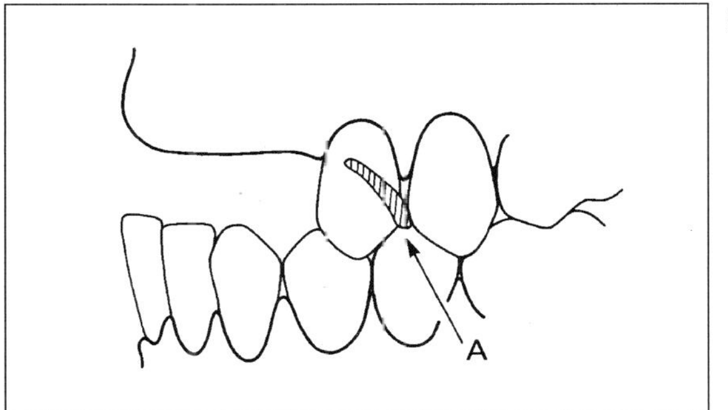

Fig **87** A circumferential retainer on 24 with a distal approach is often contra-indicated due to probable tight occlusal contact at point A.

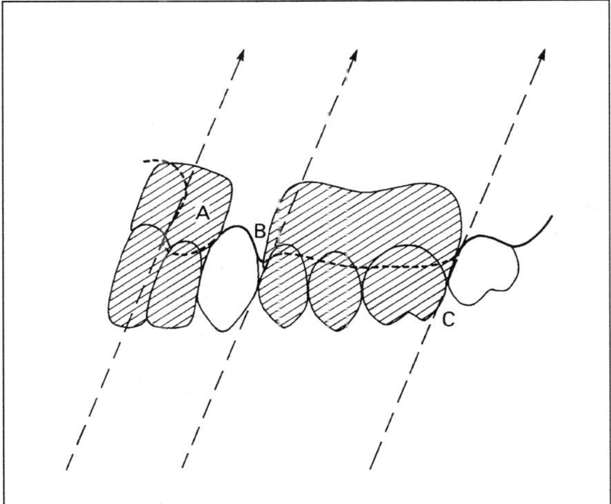

Fig **88** A denture base in a mesial undercut (A) acts as a direct retainer when the oblique path of insertion is used. It resists downward displacement of the denture at right angles to the occlusal plane.

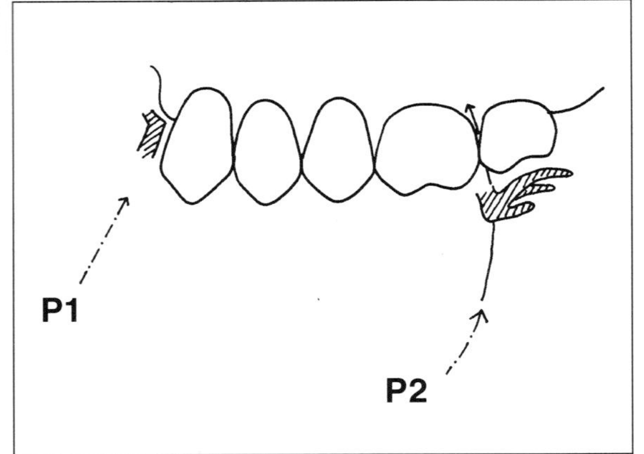

Fig **89** The rotational path of insertion changes from P1 to P2.

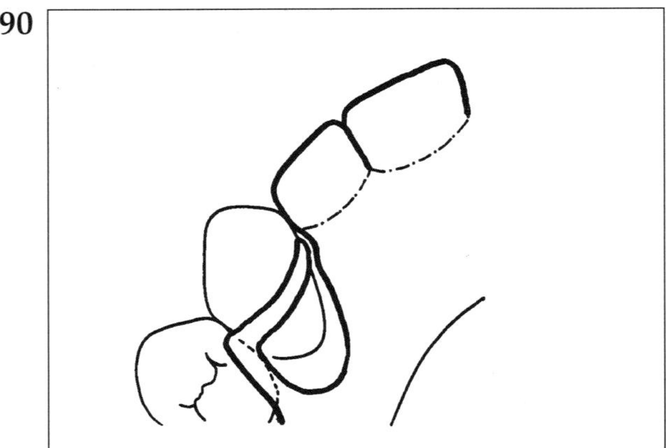

Fig **90** The retainer from the palatal aspect is utilising the mesial undercut. One disadvantage of this method is the 'little window' created on the palatal of the abutment.

Use a rotational path of insertion which works on the same principle of the denture base itself acting as a retainer in the mesial undercut. Rotational means insertion on a series of arcs derived from variable radii as the denture approaches its final seating (Fig 89).

A rotational path of insertion for anterior bases can only be used where:

- There are good mesial undercuts on the anterior abutments.
- There are no posterior edentulous areas to be restored.
- The distance between the anterior base and the posterior retentive units is great enough for rotation to occur.

Use the mesial undercut from the palatal aspect (Fig **90**).

Indirect retention

Consider Fig **91**. Assume that some form of direct retention has been found at or near the edentulous area at A and B. The base will tend to rotate at fulcrum F between A and B.

ROTATION TOWARDS X

To stop rotation towards X, you would ideally need indirect retention at point C.

A *compromise* could be extension of the denture base over point C. This compromise sacrifices optimal (tooth) support for optimal position.

Another compromise could be occlusal rests on the distal surfaces of 17 and 27. This compromise sacrifices optimal position for optimal (tooth) support.

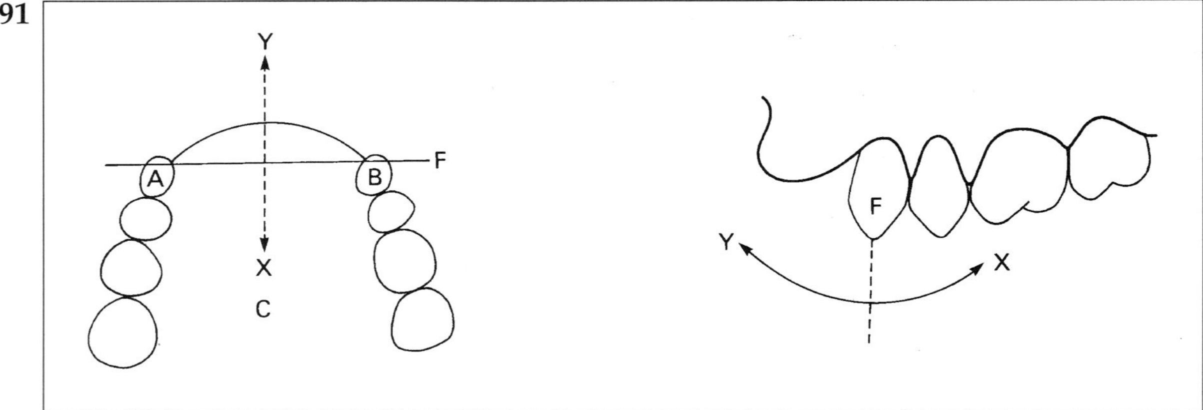

Fig **91**

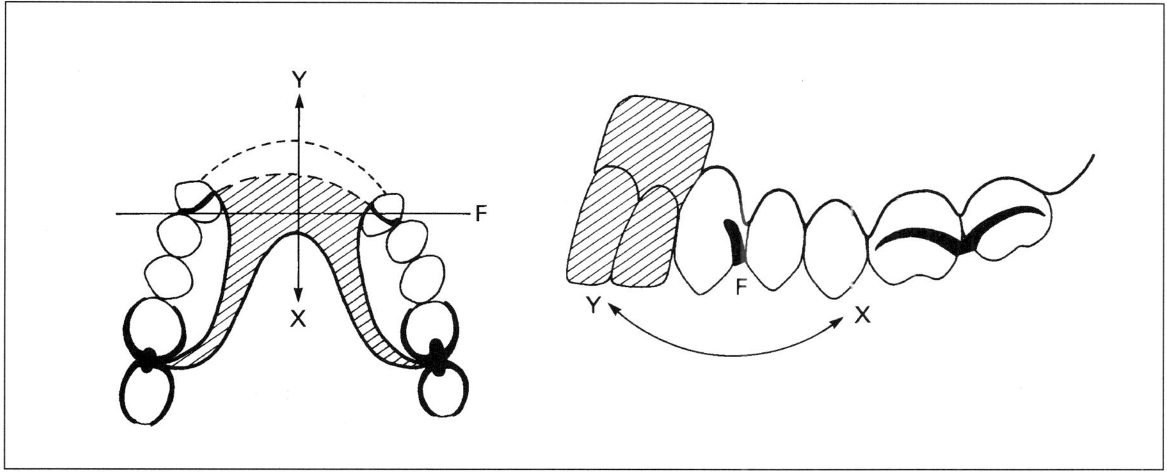

Fig **92** Rotation is around fulcrum F through the direct retainers on 13 and 23. Occlusal rests on 17, 16, 26 and 27 stop rotation towards X. Direct retention on 17 and 27 stops rotation towards Y.

ROTATION TOWARDS Y

To stop rotation towards point Y, use extra retainers at a distance from the base area.

The effectiveness of this strategy is increased by lengthening the lever arm by using the most distal teeth available (Fig **92**).

The *number of direct retainers* you need in the posterior part of the mouth will depend on the magnitude of the occlusal forces expected on the base, that is, towards Y. It may be sufficient to retain on 17 and 27 only.

Aesthetics

Problems with aesthetics with anterior dentures may be due to *compromises to achieve occlusal integrity* (see pages 43–44).

They may also be due to:

- Limitations of available space.
- Unsightly tooth undercuts.
- Awkward tissue undercuts.
- Colour matching.

AVAILABLE SPACE

The abutment teeth may have drifted or tilted into the edentulous area causing a constriction of space (Fig **93**).

Consider orthodontic correction to improve guiding surfaces and to provide space for denture teeth in edentulous areas.

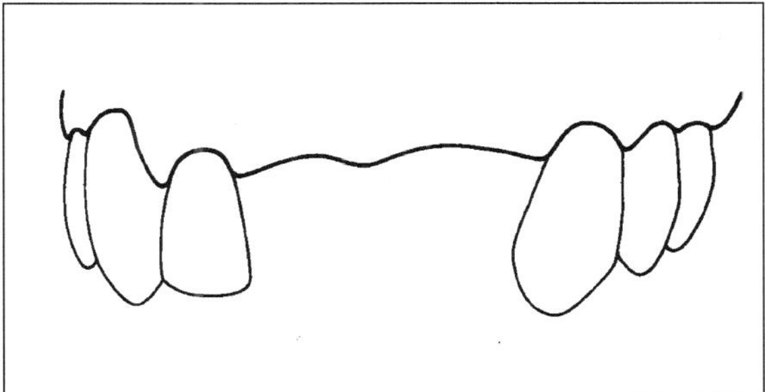

Fig **93** 12 and 23 have drifted into the space left by 11, 21 and 22.

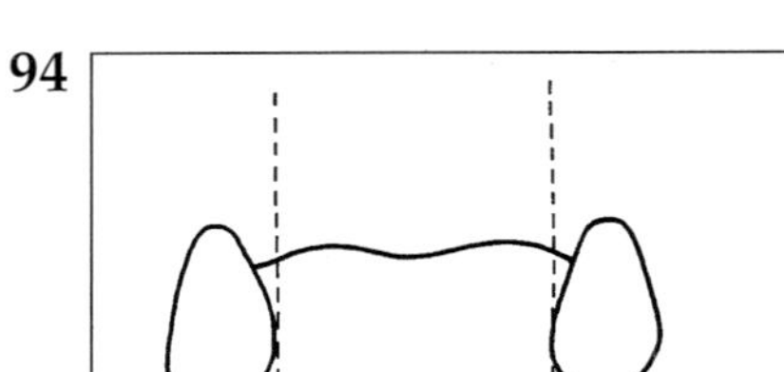

Fig **94** Setting teeth straight into a constricted space results in teeth that look too small.

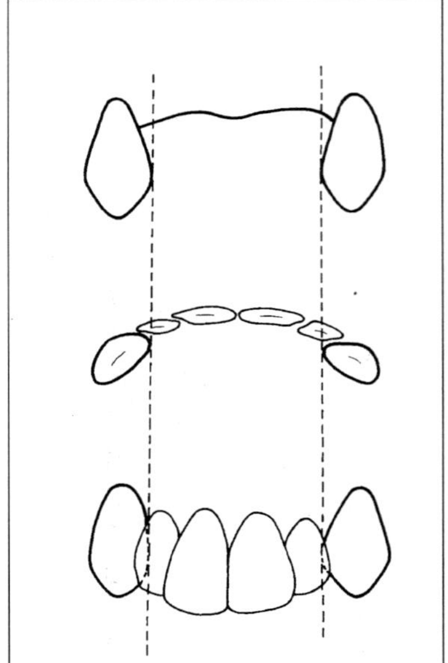

Fig **95** 13 and 23 have carefully prepared guiding planes on the mesio-labial surfaces. Teeth of the correct size are lapped to give an aesthetically pleasing result.

Fig **96** Note that the desired centre line A is not in the centre of the edentulous area. Lapping the teeth can disguise this fact.

How can you overcome this problem of space if orthodontic correction is not suitable? The best way to overcome this problem is by judicious guide plane preparation and carefully thought out lapping of artificial teeth (Figs **94**, **95**).

Always use denture teeth of the same size as the natural counterparts.

You can also use the method of guide plane preparation and tooth lapping to disguise uneven spaces which would result in an unsightly centre line (Fig **96**).

Undesirable undercuts on the mesial aspect of the abutment teeth look particularly ugly if the denture has a flange (Fig **97**).

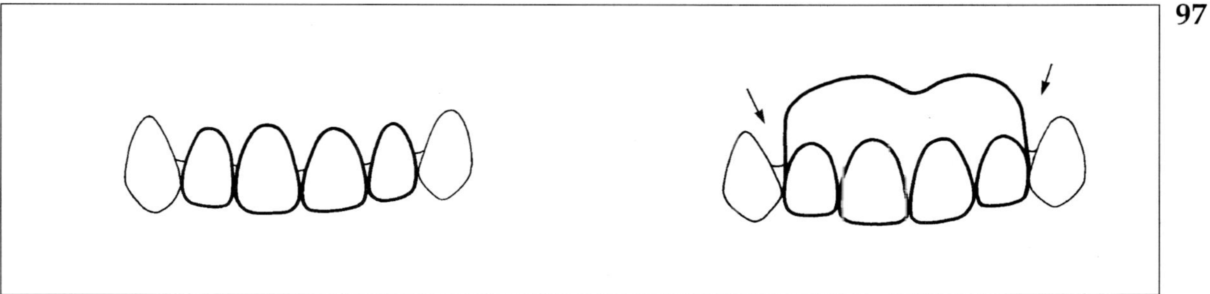

Fig **97** Gum-fitted incisors (left); the flange accentuates unsightly undercuts on the mesial aspect of 13 and 23 (right).

Even when a flange is necessary to restore lost tissue contour, you can mitigate the problem by:

- Modifying the abutment tooth surface to decrease the undercut where tooth anatomy permits.
- Using an oblique or rotational path of insertion (see pages 45 and 46) so that the undercut is filled with denture base material. Use a wide labial flange chamfered to a knife-edge lying on non-resorbed tissue. Match the acrylic flange to the colour and texture of the patient's mucosa (Fig **98**).
- Preparing mesio-labial guide planes on the canines and lapping the laterals over them so that the undercut is hidden (Fig **99**).

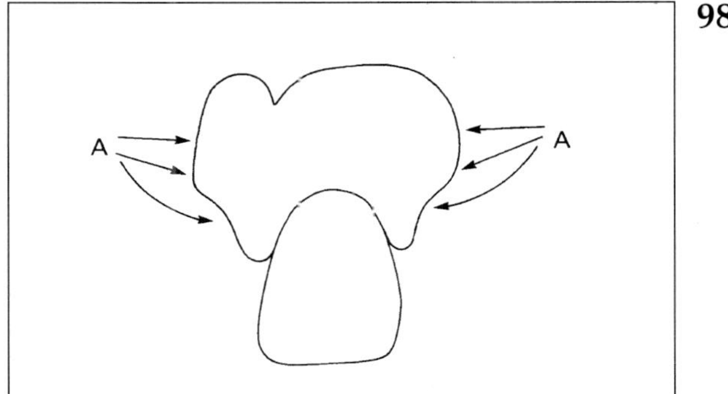

Fig **98** A wide acrylic flange replacing a central incisor. The acrylic is designed to replace lost tissue. The edges of the flange are chamfered to a knife-edge to merge with the attached mucosa (A).

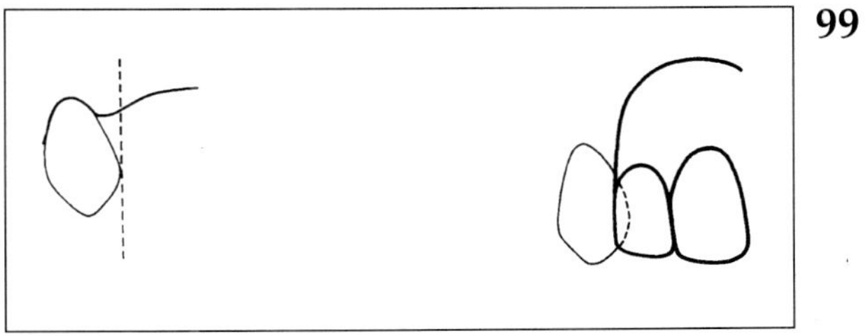

Fig **99** The undercut on the mesial aspect of 13 is hidden by the labial placement of 12, together with a wide labial flange.

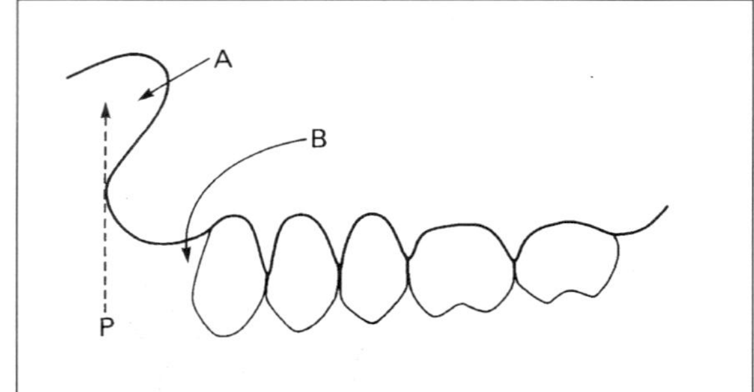

Fig **100** The conventional path of insertion (P) creates a large tissue undercut at A and B.

Anterior edentulous areas very often have large tissue undercuts which you will have to consider when deciding on a path of insertion (Fig **100**).

If possible, try to change the path of insertion to minimise such undercuts (Fig **101**)

What should you do if you cannot eliminate the tissue undercut by varying the path of insertion? Where the undercut cannot be negotiated, plan to gum-fit the teeth or to finish the flange at the height of the contour (Fig **102**).

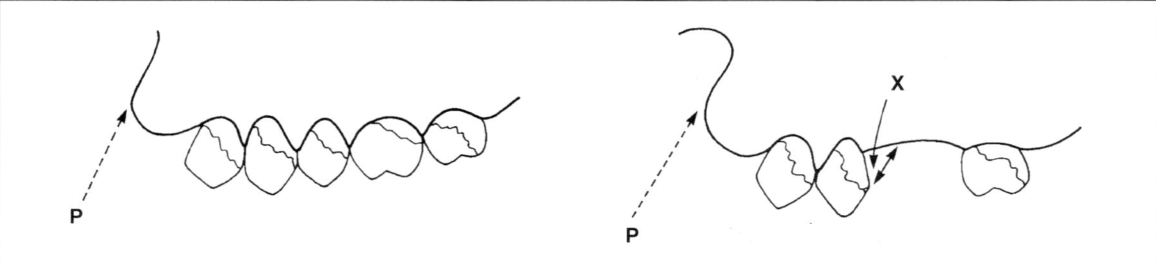

Fig **101** The path of insertion (P) is changed to eliminate the anterior tissue undercut (left); the variation of the path of insertion in this case will create an untenable undercut on the distal aspect of 25 (X) (right).

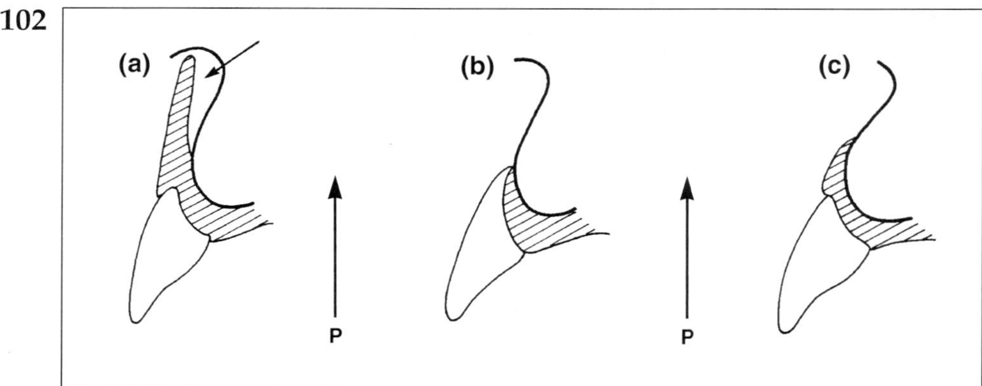

Fig **102** The path of insertion (P) creates a large tissue undercut. A flange with a gap underneath (a) is not acceptable. Either gum-fit the teeth (b), or finish the flange as a feather edge at the height of contour (c).

It is often a challenge to match the beauty, depth and variation of colour of the natural teeth.

If possible, choose tooth colour in bright daylight. Take your patient close to the window and turn off the (yellow) operating light. Fluorescent ceiling lights simulate daylight more closely.

If in doubt, choose slightly darker teeth. They will tend to become lighter if you have to grind the backs to make them fit (Fig 103). Darker teeth are also less obtrusive than lighter ones.

Use teeth of *different colours*. Most natural dentitions display a range of colours. Varying the colours of denture teeth can help them to blend together.

Modify the colour by changing the colour of the acrylic behind the tooth with, for example, amalgam powder, yellow cement or acrylic paints.

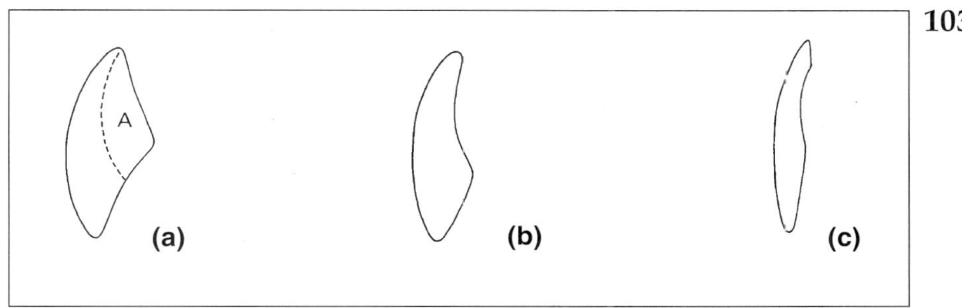

Fig 103 (a) An unground acrylic tooth. A is where the bulk of the colour is in most acrylic teeth. (b) A ground tooth. Most of the colouring acrylic has been lost and the tooth looks lighter. (c) An excessively ground tooth allows the grey of the metal backing and/or the blackness of the oral cavity to show through. In such cases, use an opaquer.

Recapitulation

- Choose your path of insertion carefully and with due regard to tissue undercuts.
- Find some direct retention close to the edentulous areas.
- Add enough direct retention far away from the edentulous areas to mitigate the problems of occlusal loading and indirect retention.
- Plan tooth modification to improve aesthetics where necessary.

PART II

Introduction

At a meeting of the Australian Prosthodontic Society, ten members were asked to devise treatment plans and denture designs for a particular patient with casts, history and radiographs provided. This exercise resulted in 13 different proposals, each hotly defended and each, on close inspection, a valid and logical scheme (Graham and Beckett, 1986).

At a meeting of the British Society for the Study of Prosthetic Dentistry, 79 prosthodontists were given identical casts of the same patient and asked to design a mandibular RPD. No design was duplicated in every detail although there were many similarities; for example, 91 per cent placed a mesial rest on the abutment tooth of DEBs (Walter, 1989).

In a similar study Frantz (1975) reported the variations in a maxillary RPD design by 57 dentists. All 57 designs of this case were different.

In 1983 Cotmore *et al.* highlighted the differences between two dental schools in the general trends in treatment and in RPD designs, and McKinstry *et al.* (1989) commented on the problems of dental students when called upon to design RPD frameworks.

Owall and Taylor (1989) noted differences in designs in different countries and commented that 'The reasons for these differences are obscure and ... such variations are difficult to explain from clinical or scientific viewpoints.'

In other words, there is rarely one 'correct' answer to the problems presented by a particular case and different dentists will be influenced by their own philosophy. We have, therefore, presented different solutions in a number of the following cases, and still other designs could also be appropriate.

This does not mean, however, that anything is acceptable. All our treatment plans and designs follow closely the guidelines set out in Part I of this text and, in the light of these guidelines, we have given our reasons for the designs proposed.

We have also included designs for two patients with examples of what is patently 'incorrect'. Such errors are not merely a matter of philosophy. They are mistakes which would seriously jeopardise the success of treatment. To be able to recognise these mistakes is the first step in understanding the basic rules of treatment planning and denture design.

'Incorrect' designs are represented on pages 151–155. There are at least five intentional mistakes in each of the designs shown.

You will note that most designs need some tooth modification. Where this involves gold or gold-based restorations, the preparations can radically alter the shape of the tooth to a more desirable form. However, where tooth modification is in enamel, it is almost always necessary to make compromises. The 'ideal' preparation must be modified to give a smooth, rounded result which blends with the natural tooth anatomy. Preparation is kept to a minimum, enamel must never be penetrated and all cut surfaces must be polished and treated with topical fluoride.

History and Examination of a Patient

A comprehensive history and examination will enable you to see the patient as a person, so that treatment planning can be geared to that person's specific wants and needs.

We have found that the following checklist helps us in gathering this information:

1 Name of patient:
2 Sex:
3 Date of birth:
4 Address and telephone number:
5 Occupation:
6 Marital status:
7 Number and ages of children:
8 Name, address and telephone number of:
    family doctor:
    family dentist:
9 Referral source:
10 Complaining of (present complaint in patient's own words):
11 History of present complaint:
12 Past dental history:
13 Past medical history (including any present problem and medication):
14 Social habits (smoking, alcohol, sports, housing, family problems, financial, job, hobbies):
15 On examination
    extra-oral (mainly signs):
    intra-oral:
      teeth present:
      dentures *in situ*:
      occlusion:
      dentures *extra situm*:
      oral hygiene:
      soft tissues:
      periodontal status:
      occlusion of natural teeth:
      restorations (charted):
16 Radiographic findings:
17 Provisional diagnosis:
18 Further investigations:
    further radiographs:
    routine blood:
    rinse, swabs and smears:
    biopsy:
    sialography:
    computer aided tomography:
    other:
19 *Definitive diagnosis:*
20 *Treatment plan:*
    referral to another:
    disposition:
21 Prognosis:
22 Fee status:

Specimen Prescription Forms
(Laboratory Sheets)

LABORATORY INSTRUCTION CARD

Patient: *Smith* .... Technician *John L.* ....

Date submitted *19.1.93* .... Date required *27.1.93*

MAJOR CONNECTOR: Maxilla .... Mandible *Lingual Bar* ....

TOOTH	37	34	33	45
Rest area	M	M	C	D
Retainer type	Ring	L - Bar	—	circumf.
Retention area	DL ·02"	MB ·01"	—	ML ·01"
Reciprocation	Self recip.	Ling. plate	—	Buccal arm
Guide plate	M	D	—	—
TOOTH	46			
Rest area	M			
Retainer type	circumf. ·01"			
Retention area	DL			
Reciprocation	Buccal arm			
Guide plate	—			

Clinical limitations *Avoid frenum buccal of 34* ....

Special instructions *Note Retention 45, 46 is on LINGUAL* ....

Signature ....

LABORATORY INSTRUCTION CARD

Patient: _Smith._ Technician: _John L._

Date submitted: _20.1.93_ Date required: _22.1.93_

MAJOR CONNECTOR: Maxilla _Mid Palatal Plate_ Mandible _________

TOOTH	17	13	23	25
Rest area	M	C	C	D
Retainer type	circumf.	i bar	—	—
Retention area	DB ·01"	DB ·01"	—	—
Reciprocation	palatal arm	cing. rest	—	—
Guide plate	M	D	D	M + D
TOOTH	27			
Rest area	M			
Retainer type	short ring			
Retention area	DB ·02"			
Reciprocation	pal. of clasp			
Guide plate	M			

Clinical limitations: _—_

Special instructions: _Post in 24 edent area._

Signature: _Aros S_

Patient No 1 (Figs 106–132)

History and examination

Name: A.C.W.
Sex: female
Age: 42 years
Occupation: housewife
c/o: present partial upper denture feels loose; wondering about need for lower denture
PDH: last seen by dentist about a year ago; teeth extracted because of caries in stages since age 17 years; acrylic denture about 5 years old
PMH: none relevant
Social habits: lives active, happy, family life
o/e: never worn lower RPD; a number of restorations have leaking margins; good periodontal health; above average hygiene
Radiographs: none available

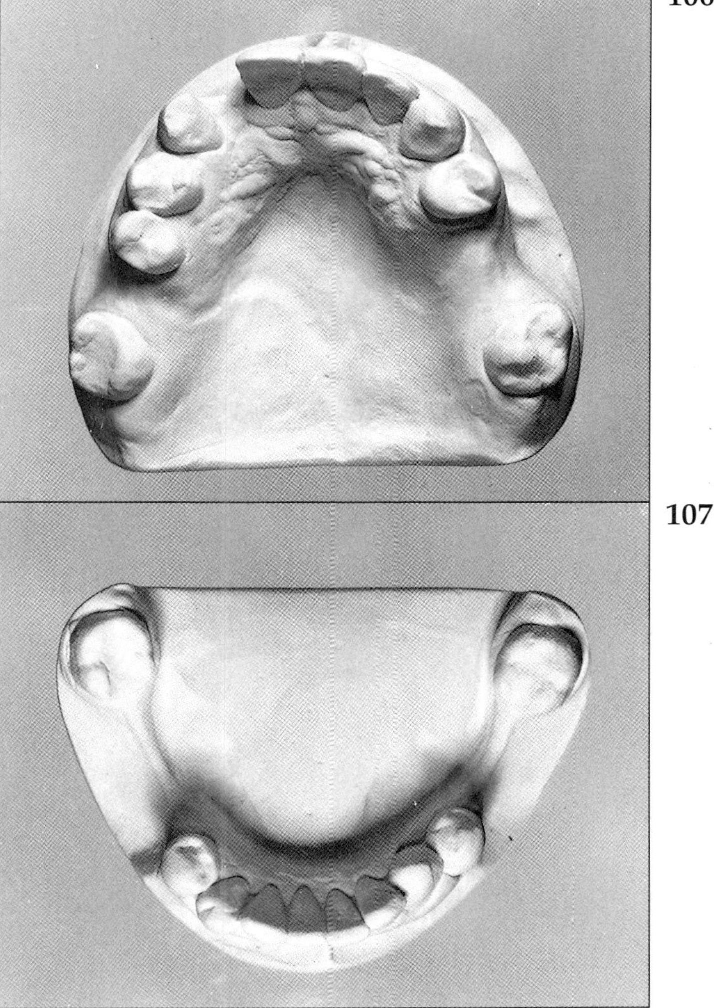

106

107

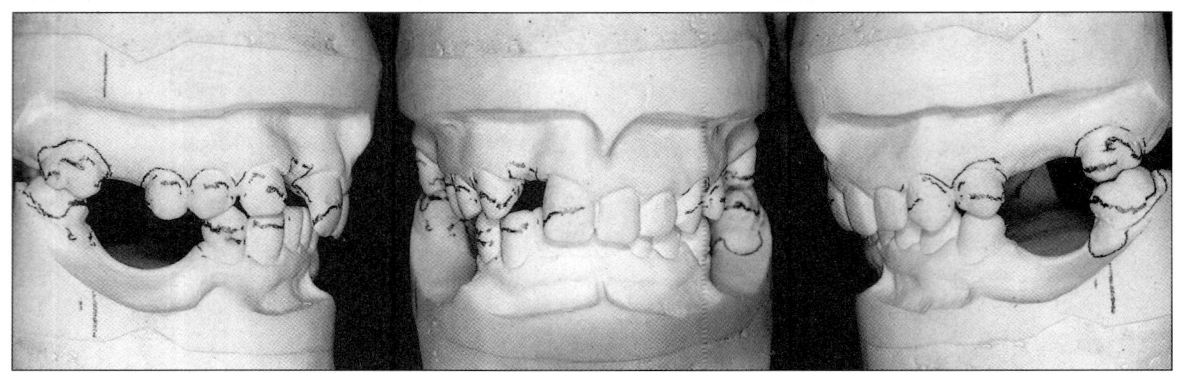

108
109
110

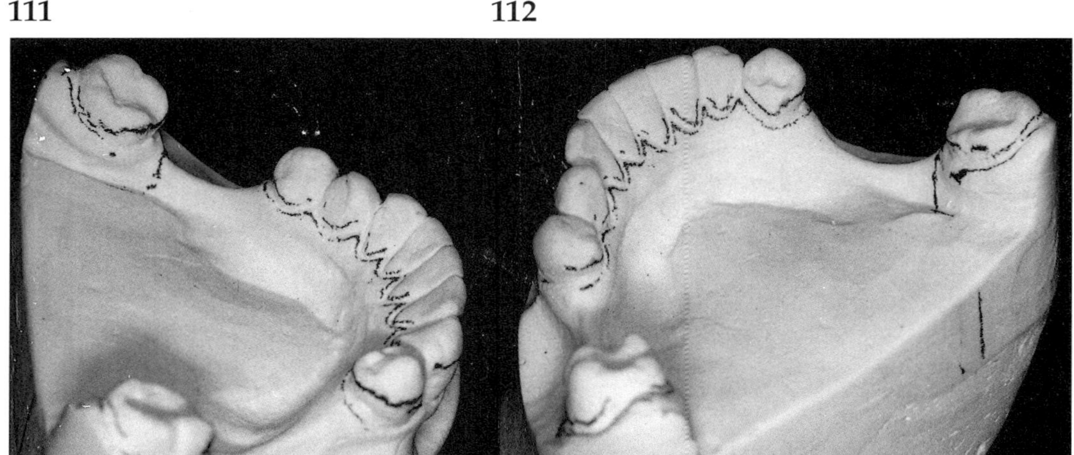

111
112

Treatment plan

Does this patient need RPD treatment?

The patient would like 12 restored for aesthetic reasons. She also feels her cheeks are collapsing because of lower posterior tooth loss.

Dentally, some form of prosthesis is necessary to prevent the overeruption of 15. Other prosthodontic restoration is not necessary unless symptoms occur.

Treatment options

MAXILLA
- FPD (bridge) 12 only.
- FPD for all edentulous areas.
- FPD to restore 12 and RPD for posterior edentulous areas.
- RPD (acrylic or metal).

MANDIBLE
- No prosthesis, if 15 is restored to function.
- FPD for both edentulous areas.
- RPD (metal).

Decision and treatment plan

This is influenced by history and finances, together with lack of full information on periodontal tissues.

- Replace restorations where necessary and ensure occlusion is stable.
- Upper and lower cobalt-chromium RPD.

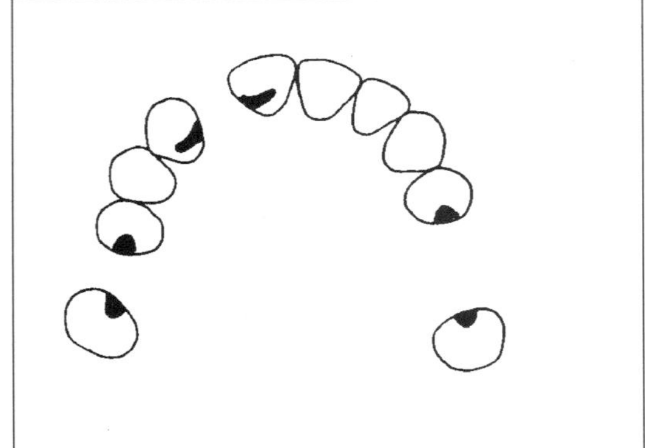

Fig **113** Support.

Design A (A.R.M.)

Maxilla

Edentulous areas to be restored
3 tooth supported.

Support
- Occlusal rests 17(M), 15(D), 24(D) and 27(M).
- Cingulum rests 13 and 11.

Retentive pattern
Triangle between 17, 27 and 24 augmented by a wide labial flange on labial of 12.

Retention
- Occlusally approaching retainers on 17 and 27 (reciprocated by plate).
- Gingivally approaching retainer on 24 (reciprocated by palatal arm).

Connector
Posterior palatal bar with right anterior strut.

Acrylic anchorage
- Post for 12 (alloy to back cingulum).
- Mesh for 16, 25 and 26.

Tooth modification
Lower survey line 27(MB) to allow the rigid shoulder of the retainer to be positioned.

Comments
The use of the wide labial flange, primarily for aesthetic reasons, aids retention in the common path of displacement, that is, at right angles to the occlusal plane. Insertion will be upwards and backwards. Survey and blocking out, particularly distal of 15 and 24, has to be done carefully.

Fig **114** Retentive pattern. R = retainers; AR = additional retention.

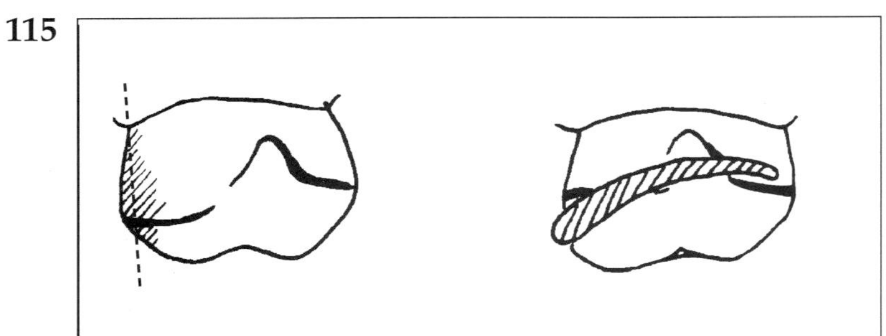

Fig **115** The survey line is lowered on the MB surface of 27 to accommodate the rigid shoulder of the retainer.

Mandible

EDENTULOUS AREAS TO BE RESTORED
2 tooth supported.

SUPPORT
Occlusal rests 37(M), 34(D), 44(D) and 47(M). The patient closed on 0.3 mm casting wax to verify adequate space for rests after preparation.

RETENTIVE PATTERN
Straight line.

RETENTION
Gingivally approaching on 34 and 44 (reciprocated by lingual arms).

CONNECTOR
Sub-lingual bar.

ACRYLIC ANCHORAGE
Mesh against fish-tail stops of sub-lingual bar.

TOOTH MODIFICATION
• Guide planes 37(M), 47(M), 34(D) and 44(D).
• Add-on composite 34(B) to provide undercut.

COMMENTS
This design lacks indirect retention which could be provided by a Kennedy bar (continuous clasp) on the lingual surface of the incisors. Alternatively, retainers could be placed on 37 or 47, but angulation and survey lines are not favourable. The suggested design has the benefit of simplicity.

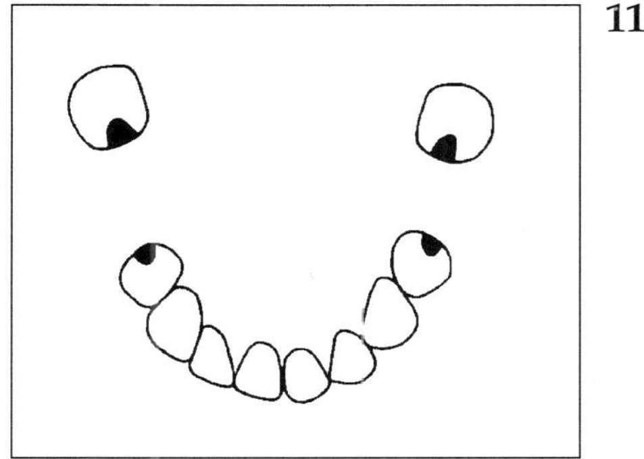

Fig **116** Support.

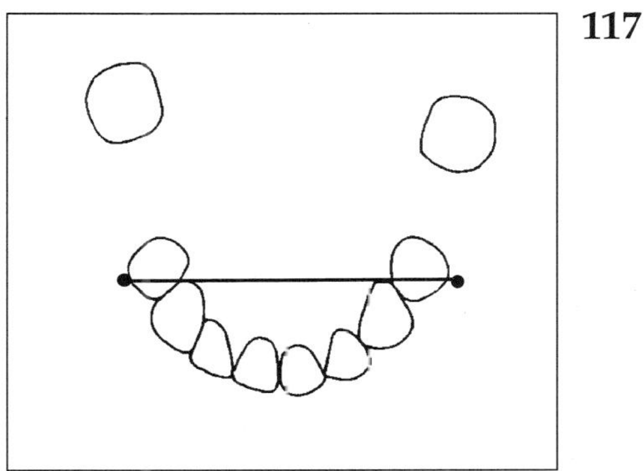

Fig **117** Retentive pattern.

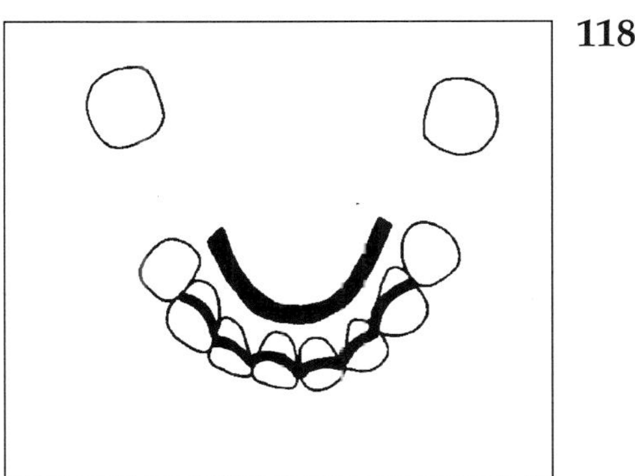

Fig **118** The continuous clasp would provide indirect retention, but often irritates the tongue.

119

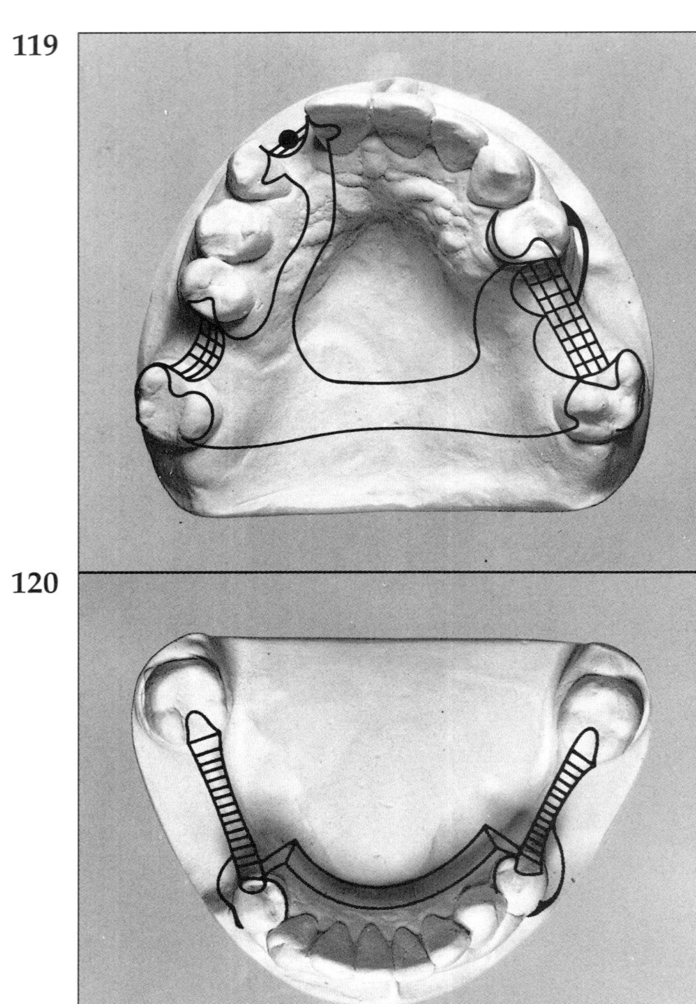

120

Design B (S.K.L.)

Maxilla

EDENTULOUS AREAS TO BE RESTORED
3 tooth supported.

SUPPORT
* Occlusal rests 17(M), 15(M) and (D), 24(D) and 27(M).
* Cingulum rest 13 and 11.

RETENTIVE PATTERN
Triangle between 17, 24 and 27 augmented by guide planes on proximal aspects of all abutments.

RETENTIVE UNITS:
* 17 and 27 shortened ring clasps from palatal into DB undercuts (self-reciprocating).
* 24 circumferential into the MP undercut (reciprocated by an extended guide plane on to the DB surface).

CONNECTOR
Mid-palatal plate with anterior strut.

ACRYLIC ANCHORAGE
* Post for 12.
* Mesh for 16, 25 and 26.

TOOTH MODIFICATION
Smooth occlusal rest areas 17(M), 15(M) and (D), 24(D) and 27(M). Guide planes on all proximal surfaces.

COMMENTS
The shortened ring clasps on 17 and 27 make efficient use of existing survey lines, and are aesthetic.

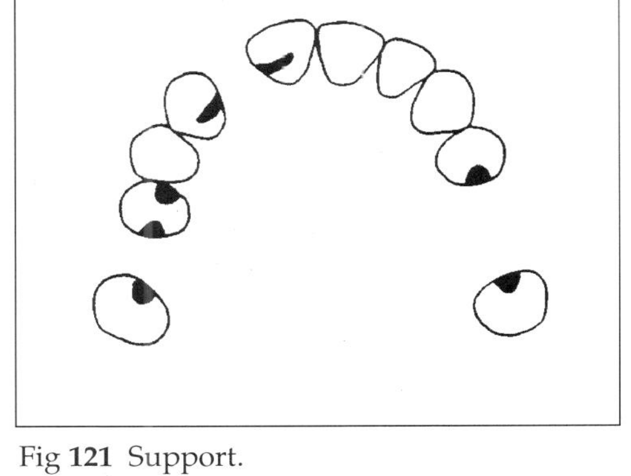

Fig **121** Support.

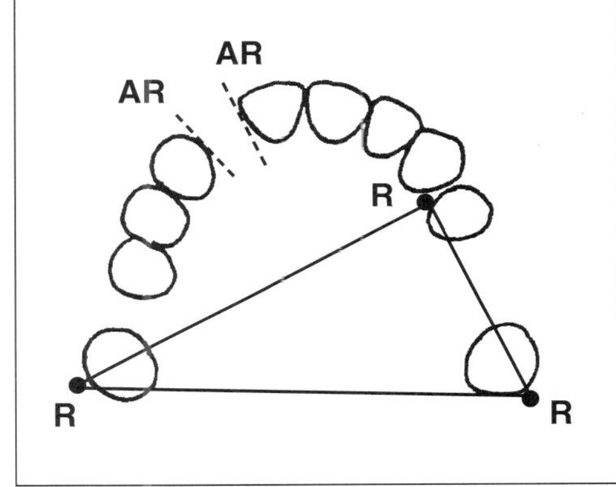

Fig **122** Retentive pattern.

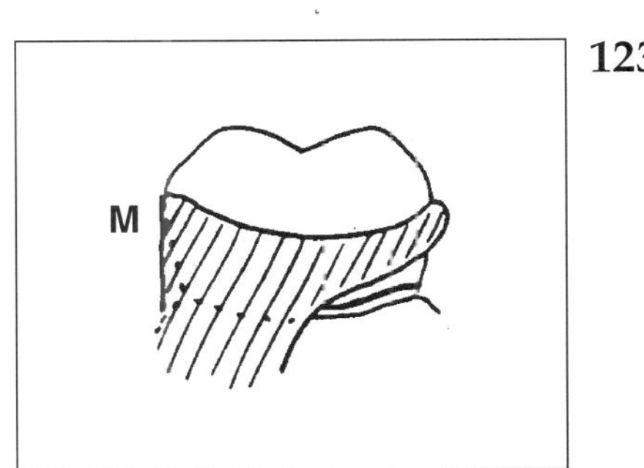

Fig **123** Shortened ring clasp on 17, palatal.

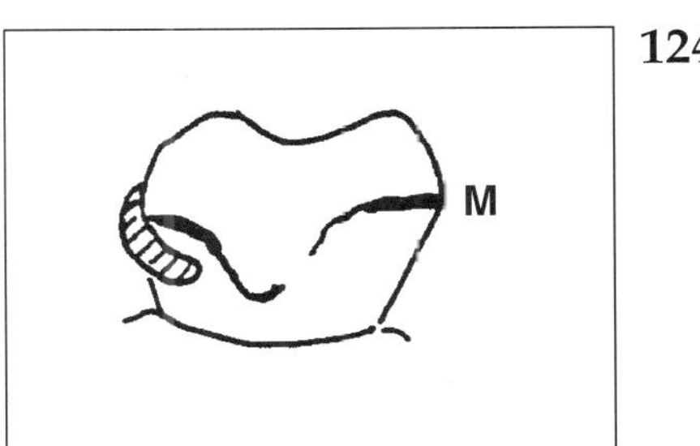

Fig **124** Shortened ring clasp on 17, buccal.

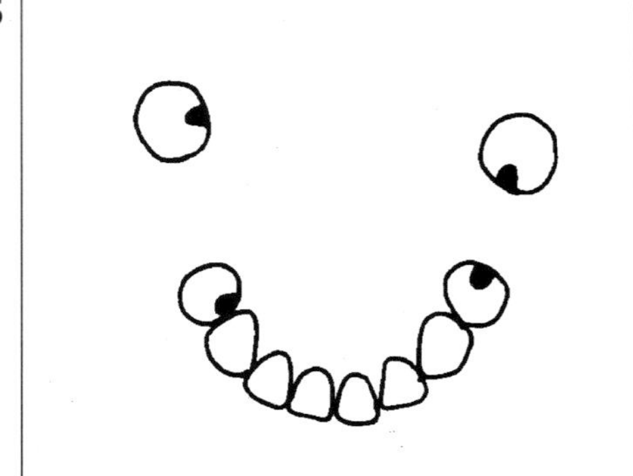

Fig **125** Support.

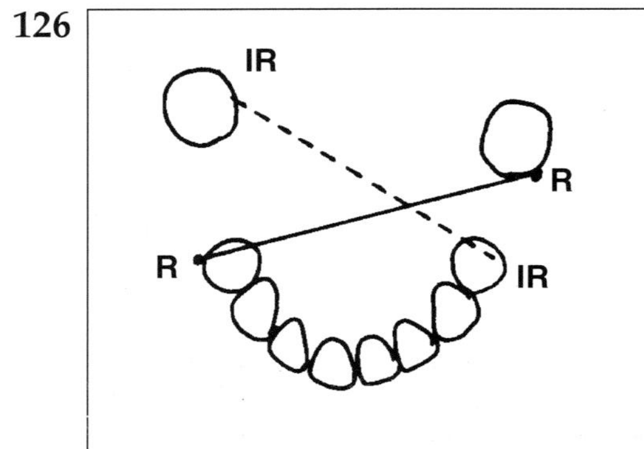

Fig **126** Retentive pattern.

Mandible

Edentulous areas to be restored
2 tooth supported.

Support
Occlusal rests 37(M), 34(D), 44(M) and 47(ML).

Retentive pattern
Straight line between 37 and 44 augmented by occlusal rests on 34 and 47 (which act as indirect retention) and guide planes on all proximal surfaces.

Retentive units
• 37 inverted C-clasp utilising MB undercut reciprocated by lingual arm.
• 44 I-bar into DB undercut reciprocated by lingual plate.

Connector
Lingual bar.

Tooth modification
• Smooth occlusal rest areas, 37(M), 34(D), 44(M) and 47(ML).
• Lower survey line 37(MB) for the rigid part of the retainer and lingual (for rigid reciprocation).
• Guide planes on all proximal surfaces.

Comments
• Rests on 44 and 47 would ideally be placed on 44(D) and 47(M). The position of the rests has been moved to avoid interfering with the occlusion.
• Angulation on 37 and 47 is not really favourable for retention, and requires substantial tooth modification to accommodate the rigid portions of the retainer arm and the rigid reciprocating arm.

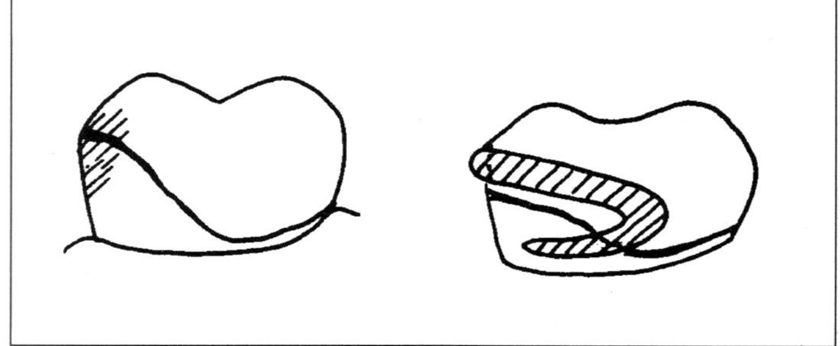

Fig **127** Tooth modification is necessary to accomodate the rigid shoulder of the retainer.

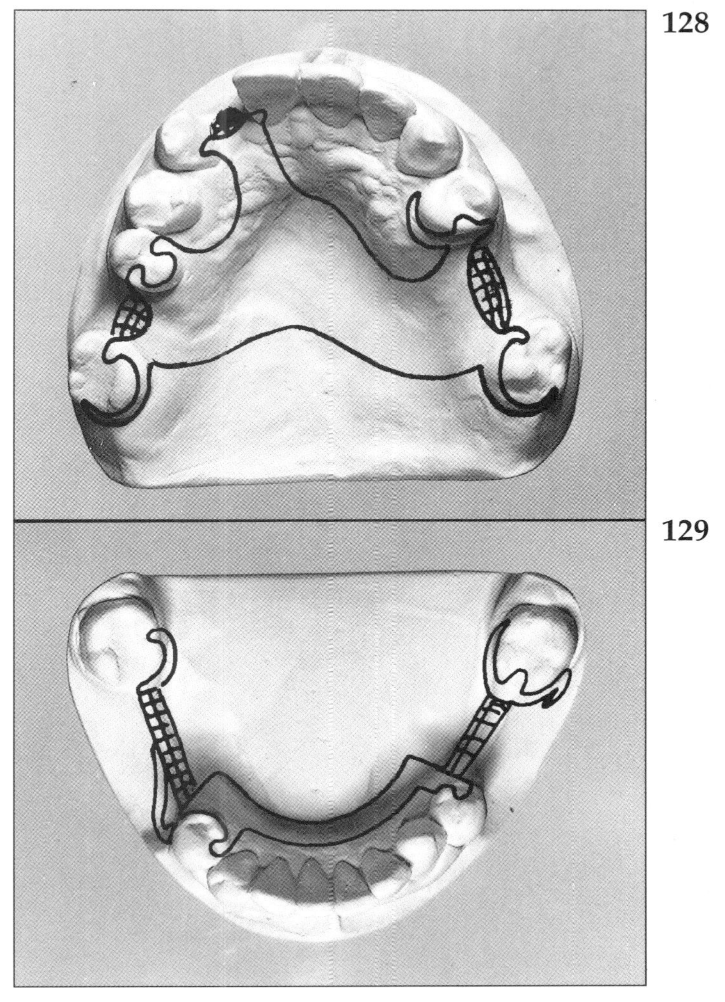

128

129

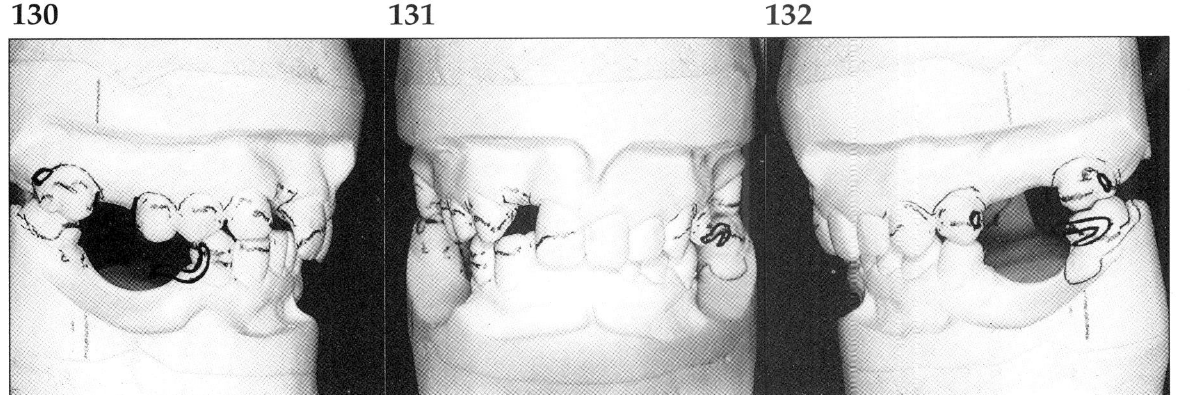

130   131   132

Patient No 2 (Figs 133–152)

History and examination

Patient 2: E.B.T.   *Sex:* male

Age: 46 years   *Occupation:* railway porter

c/o: present acrylic dentures are reasonably comfortable, but lower denture recently fractured in the midline

PDH: dentures made 18 months ago; teeth extracted because of caries and 'gum disease'

PMH: none relevant

o/e: early marginal gingivitis (palatal and lingual); teeth caries free; hygiene fair

Radiographs: full mouth intra-oral

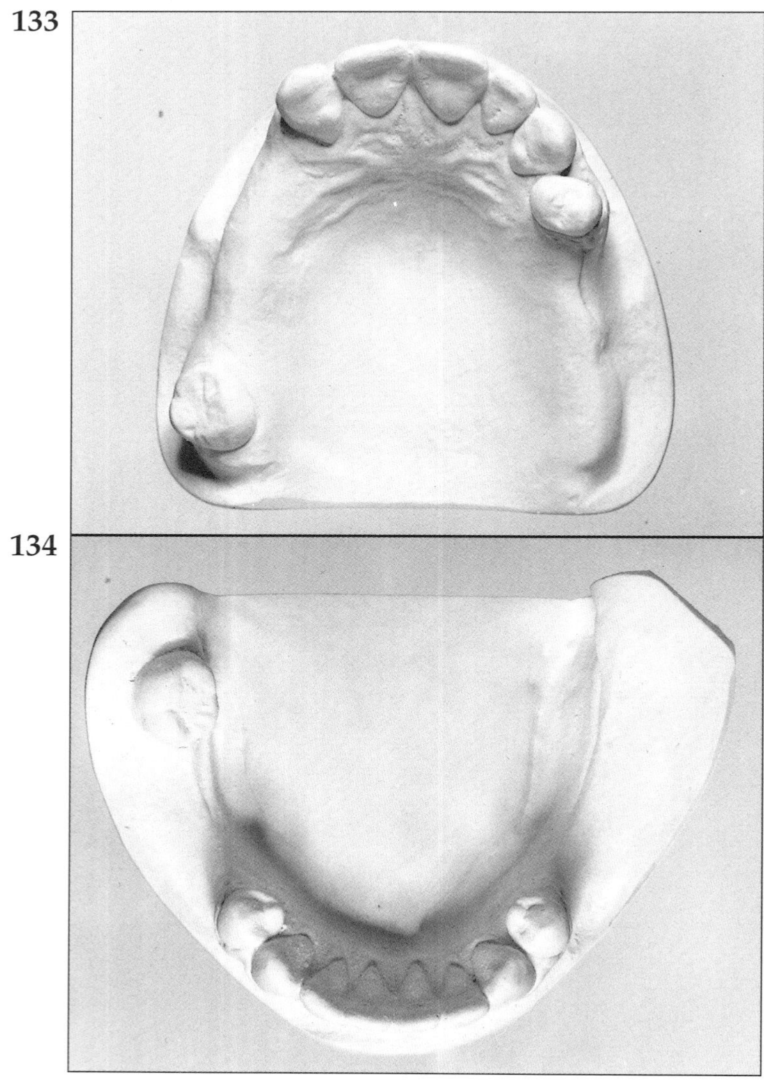

133

134

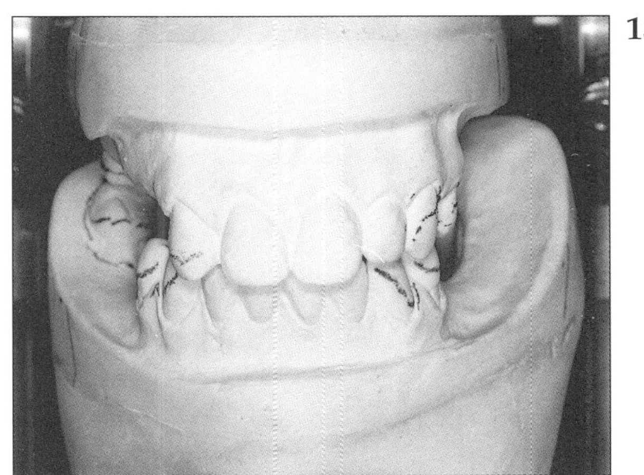

135

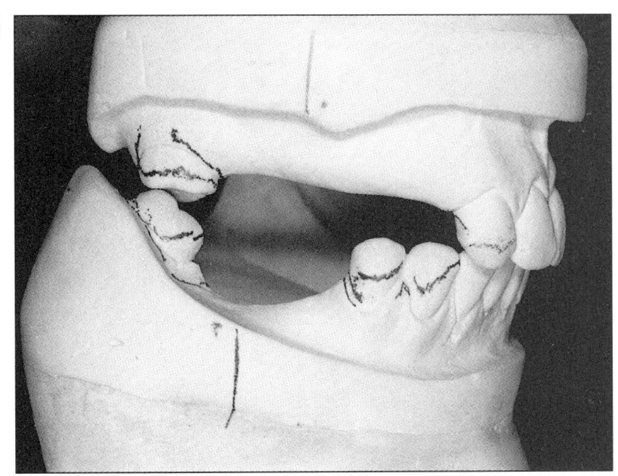

136

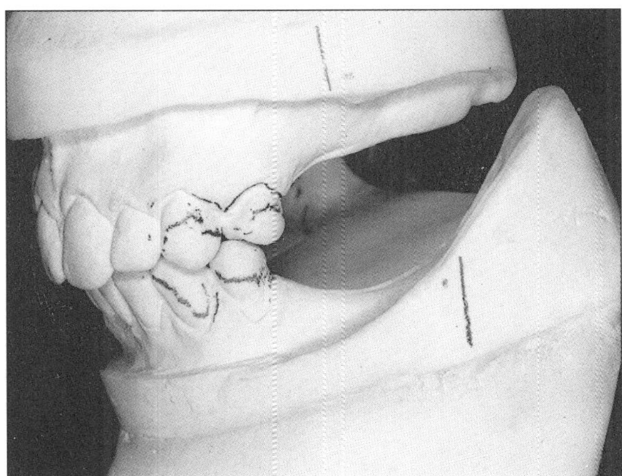

137

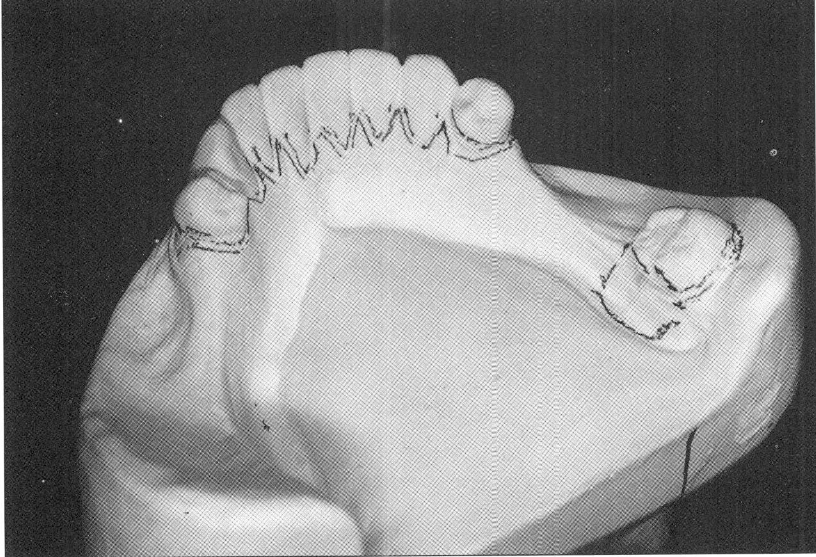

138

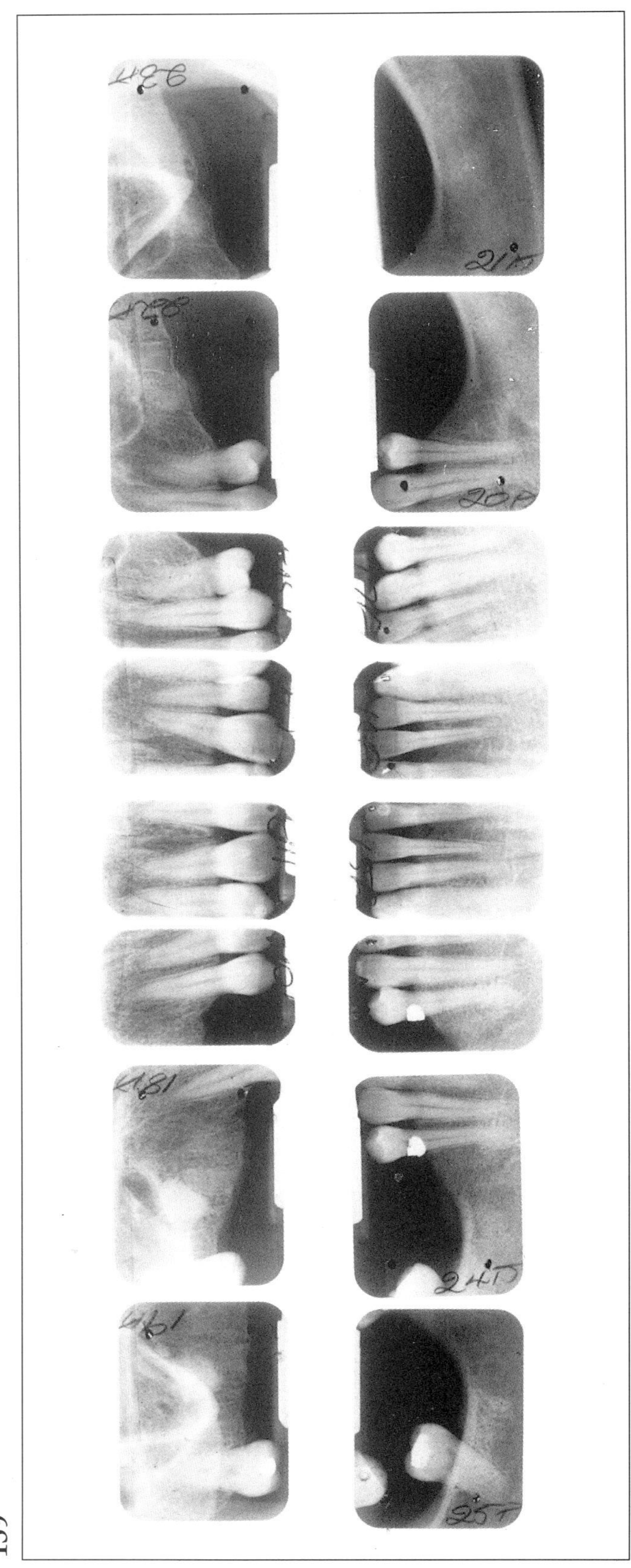

139

Treatment plan

Does this patient need RPD treatment?

The patient would like a denture for aesthetic reasons and to improve mastication.

Dentally, there is insufficient posterior support:

- 48 is not locked in occlusion and is likely to drift and tilt mesially.
- 24 could drift distally and lose its positive occlusal stop.

Treatment options

- RPD (metal or acrylic).
- Osseointegrated implants (if bone and finances permit).

Decision and treatment plan

This is influenced by the patient's wishes and good bone support. The decision is also influenced by the poor response to the previous (acrylic) RPD which was a possible cause of the patient's gingivitis, and which broke.

- Oral hygiene instruction.
- Retained root upper right quadrant; no pathology; patient informed; leave.
- Cobalt-chromium upper and lower RPD.

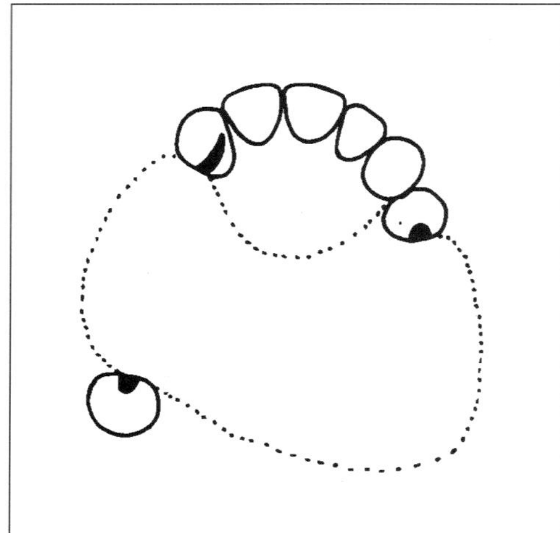

Fig **140** Support.

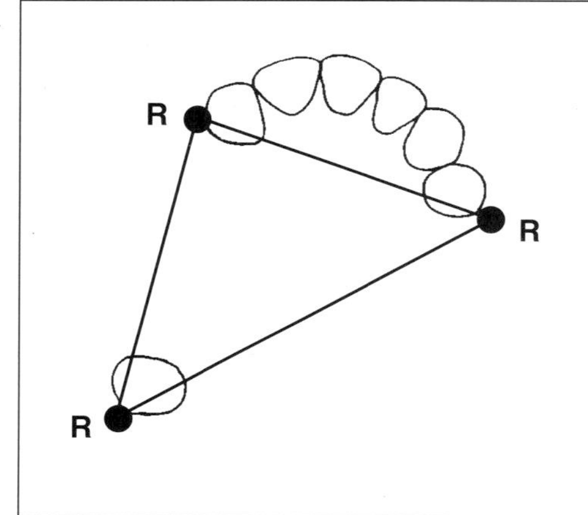

Fig **141** Retentive pattern.

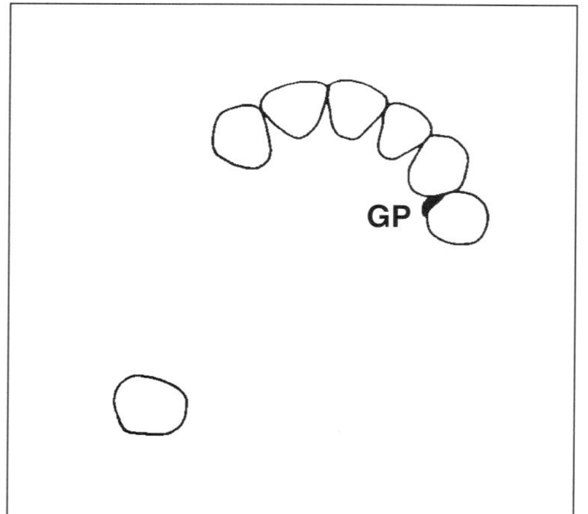

Fig **142** The guide plane on the ML surface stops the distal movement of the base.

Design

Maxilla

Edentulous areas to be restored
1 tooth supported.
1 tooth and mucosa supported.

Support
- Occlusal rests 18(M) and 24 (D). (The rest would normally be on the mesial aspect for a DEB. It has been changed to the distal aspect because the mesial has an occlusal stop.)
- Cingulum rest 13.
- Maximum tissue coverage of distal extension saddle area.

Retentive pattern
Triangle between 18, 13 and 24.

Retentive units
- 18 ring clasp into DB undercut (self-reciprocating). (*See* page 63).
- 13 I-bar into DB undercut.
- 24 L-bar (reciprocated by palatal arm on to MP surface).

Stabilisation
Wide palatal arm on 24.
Note: the palatal arm extends to the mesial surface to stop the denture moving distally.

Connector
Wide palatal strap avoiding rugae and finishing in left hamular notch.

Tooth modification
- Smooth areas for occlusal rests and cingulum rest.
- Guide planes on proximal surfaces.
Special note: the guide plane on 24 is on the ML surface.

Mandible

EDENTULOUS AREAS TO BE RESTORED
1 tooth supported.
1 tooth and mucosa supported.

SUPPORT
- Occlusal rests on 34(M), 44(M) (the mesial surface is more expedient to simplify the addition of a cingulum arm on 43) and 48(M) (a distal rest to give added support for a ring clasp would normally be added; in this case it would interfere with the occlusion).
- Maximum tissue coverage of distal extension area.

RETENTIVE PATTERN
Triangle between 34, 44 and 48 augmented by arm on 43 (indirect retention) and guide planes on proximal surfaces.

RETENTIVE UNITS
- 34 I-bar into mid-buccal undercut (reciprocated by lingual plate).
- 44 circumferential into MB undercut (reciprocated by lingual plate).
- 48 ring clasp lying above survey line on buccal surface where the survey line is low and tucking into the DL undercut (self-reciprocating).

CONNECTOR
Lingual bar.

STABILISATION
Mesial rest on 34 prevents distal movement of the denture.

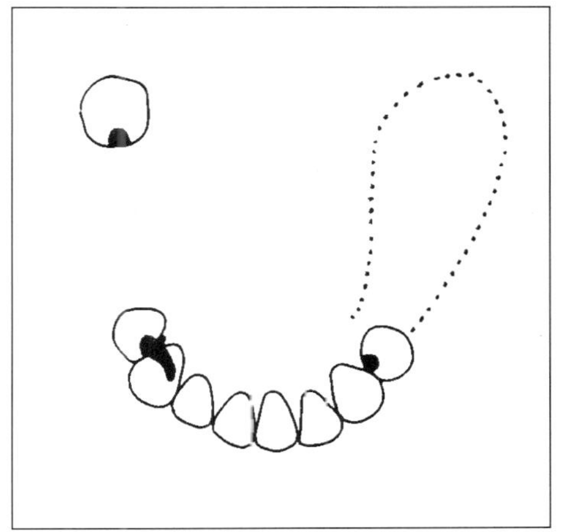

Fig **143** Support.

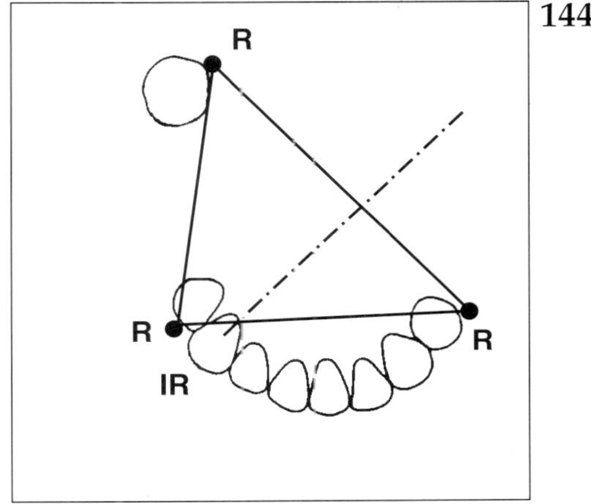

Fig **144** Retentive pattern.

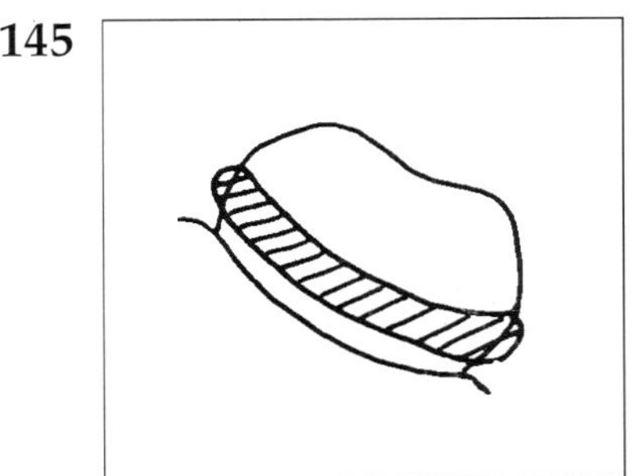

Fig **145** Ring clasp on 48 buccal surface.

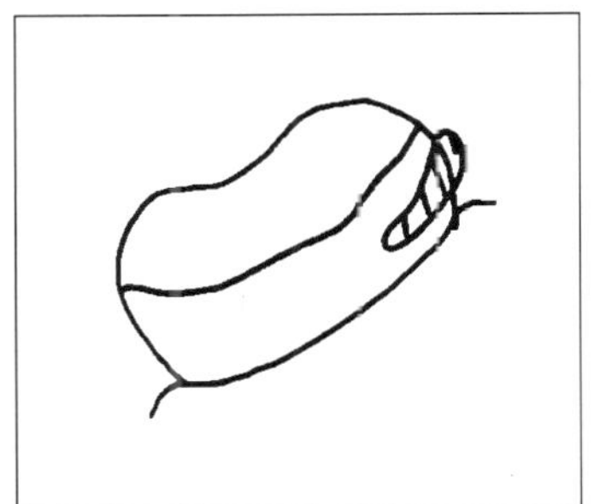

Fig **146** Ring clasp on 48 lingual surface.

147

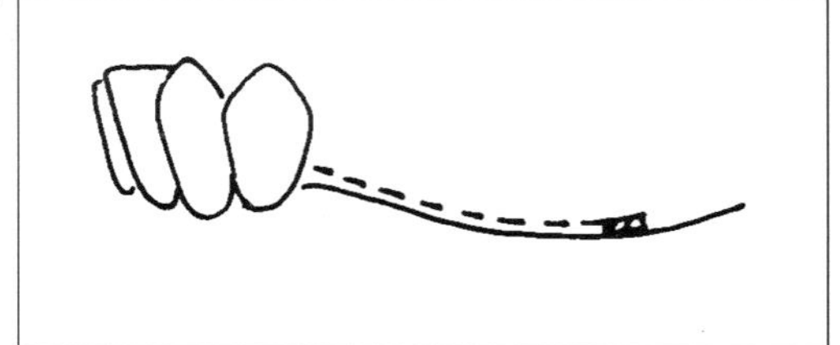

Fig 147 Mesh has a tissue stop for a DEB.

Mesh over all restored edentulous areas; tissue stop on DE area.

TOOTH MODIFICATION
- Smooth areas for occlusal rests.
- Lower survey line 48(MB).
- Guide planes 44(D) and 48(M).

COMMENTS:
The ring clasp on 48 is not ideal as the clasp is too long and liable to distort. However, any other solution would entail extensive tooth modification to lower the survey line on the lingual surface for (rigid) reciprocation of a buccal retainer, or for the first (rigid) section of a circumferential clasp. For this reason the ring clasp has been chosen here.

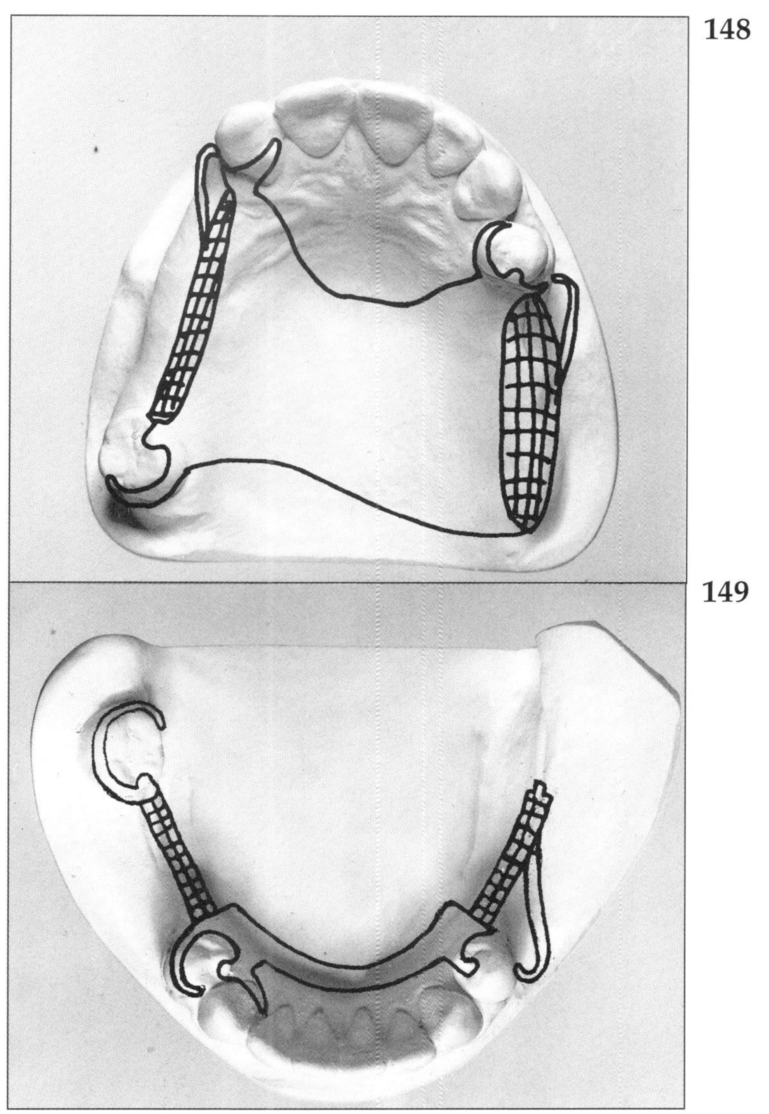

148

149

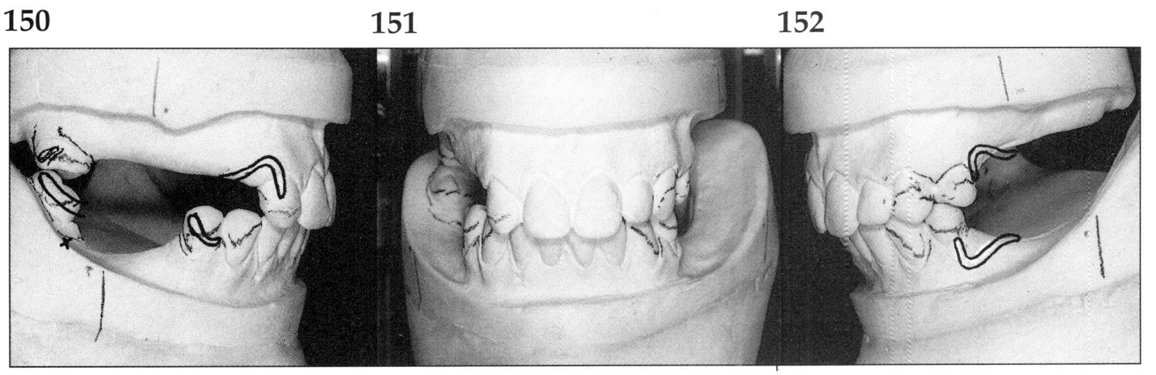

150

151

152

Patient No 3 (Figs 153–170)

History and examination

Patient 3: S.R.   *Age:* 53 years

Sex: male   *Occupation:* butcher

c/o: maxillary acrylic RPD six years old; left premolar broken off and lost; some pain biting lower right first molar

PDH: occasional fillings in the last few years; never worn lower denture

PMH: controlled diabetic

o/e: marginal gingivitis maxillary anteriors; mild palatal denture-induced hyperplasia; pain on percussion 46 (vital); cervical overhang 27; hygiene good

Radiographs: full mouth intra-oral

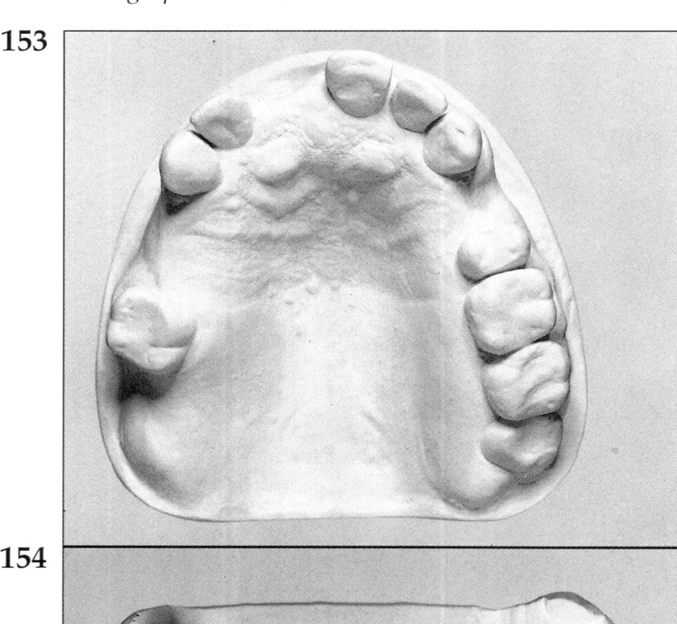

153

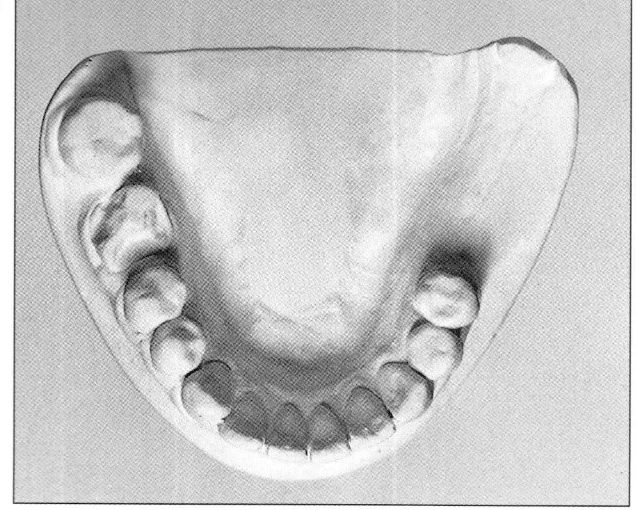

154

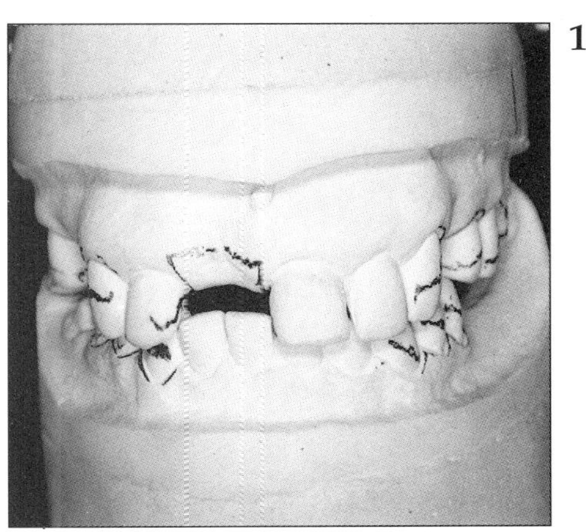

155

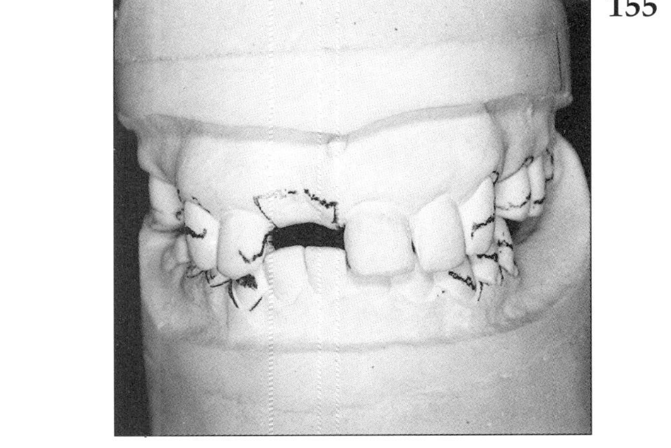

156

157

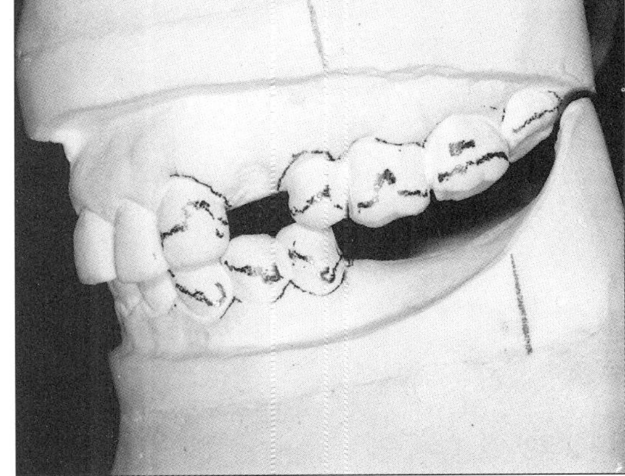

158

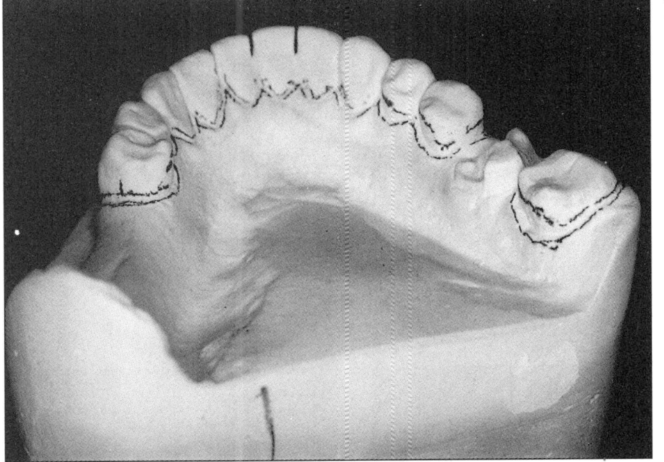

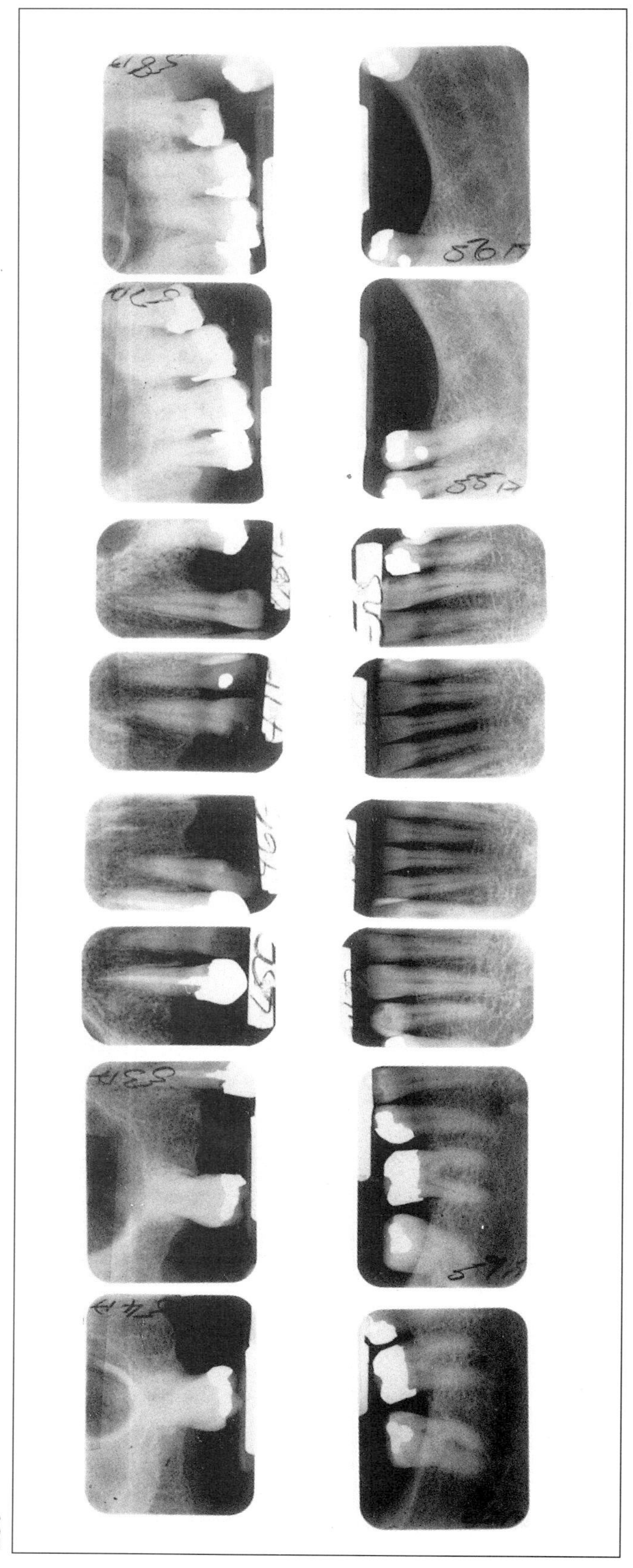

159

Treatment plan

Does this patient need RPD treatment?

The patient would like an upper denture for aesthetic reasons and a lower denture because he feels 'unbalanced'.

Dentally, a denture is necessary to prevent further overeruption of 26 and 27.

Treatment options

MAXILLA
- Restore posterior maxillary edentulous areas with fixed prostheses (difficult due to diastema), and 11 with an osseointegrated implant.
- RPD (acrylic or metal).

MANDIBLE
- Restore 46. No prosthesis.
- Restore 46. RPD (acrylic or metal).
- Extract 46. RPD (acrylic or metal).

Decision and treatment plan

This is influenced by finances, patient's wishes and bone support:

- Treat palatal hyperplasia.
- Extract 28.
- Reduce the cervical overhang on 27. Recontour the crown on 13 and restore the integrity of the margins.
- Restore 46 with a crown contoured for optimal undercuts.
- Upper and lower cobalt-chromium RPDs.

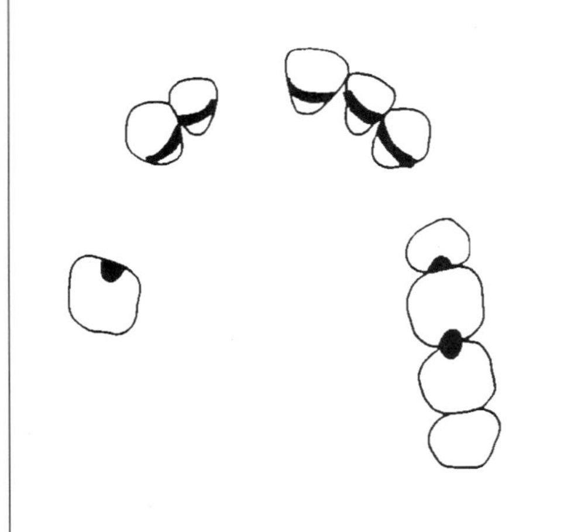

Fig **160** Support.

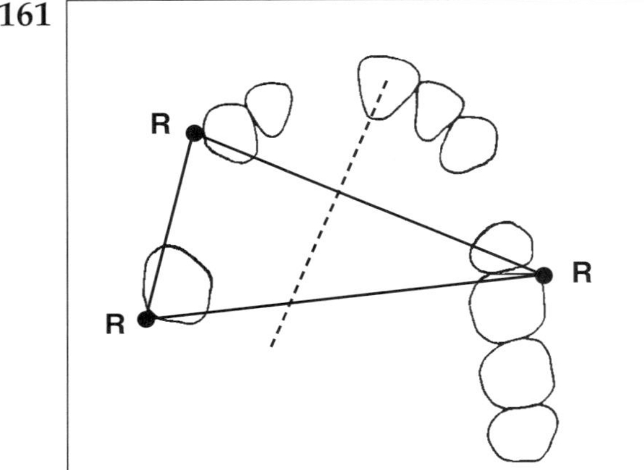

Fig **161** Retentive pattern.

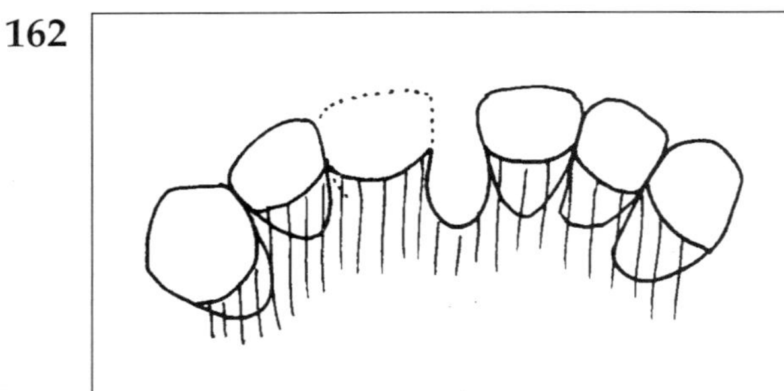

Fig **162** Connector cut away behind diastema.

Design

Maxilla

EDENTULOUS AREAS TO BE RESTORED
3 tooth supported.

SUPPORT
- Occlusal rests 16(M), 25(D), 26(D) and 27(M).
- Cingulum rests 13, 12, 21, 22 and 23.

RETENTIVE PATTERN
Triangle between 16, 13 and 26 augmented by a cingulum rest on 21 (indirect retention) and guide planes on proximals of posterior edentulous areas.

RETENTIVE UNITS
- 16 ring clasp into DB undercut (self-reciprocating).
- 13 I-bar into DB undercut (reciprocated by palatal plate).
- 26 circumferential clasp into MB undercut (reciprocated by palatal plate).

CONNECTOR
'Horseshoe' plate cut back between 11 and 21 to allow for diastema between these teeth (indicated by the size of the edentulous area in relation to the size of 21).

ACRYLIC ANCHORAGE
- Post for 11.
- Mesh for other edentulous areas.

TOOTH MODIFICATION
- Smooth occlusal rest areas.
- Lower survey line 26(DB).
- Widen embrasure between 26 and 27.
- Guide planes 16(M), 13(D), 23(D) and 25(M).
- Level incisal surface 41 and 42.

COMMENTS
Rests have been placed on 26 and 27 to stop overeruption. 13 is a doubtful abutment. Support is shared with 12. If 13 is lost the denture can be modified by adding a tooth and placing a retainer on 23. This makes a smaller, but still viable, triangle.

Mandible

EDENTULOUS AREAS TO BE RESTORED
1 tooth and mucosa supported.

SUPPORT
- Occlusal rests on 35(M) and 34(D).
- Maximum coverage of edentulous area.
- Additional rests on 45(D), 46(M) and 47(L) to give cross-arch stabilisation.

RETENTIVE PATTERN
Straight line between 35 and 46 augmented by an additional occlusal rest on 44(M) for indirect retention.

RETENTIVE UNITS
- 35 L-bar into MB undercut (reciprocated by lingual plate).
- 46 circumferential into DB undercut (reciprocated by a very wide rigid arm on the lingual surface).

CONNECTOR
Lingual bar.

TOOTH MODIFICATION
Smooth occlusal rest areas on 35(M), 34(D), 45(D) and 47 (long L).

COMMENTS
A wide reciprocating arm on (crowned) 46 extends and becomes a long occlusal rest on the lingual surface of 47 to provide function for this tooth and avoid possible tipping and overeruption if the point contact with 16 is lost.

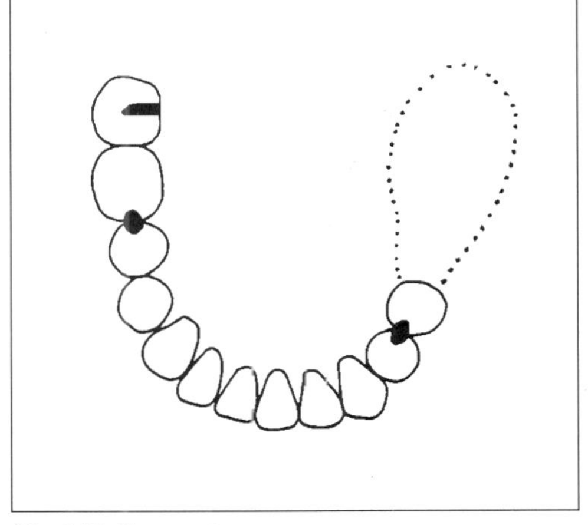

Fig **163** Support.

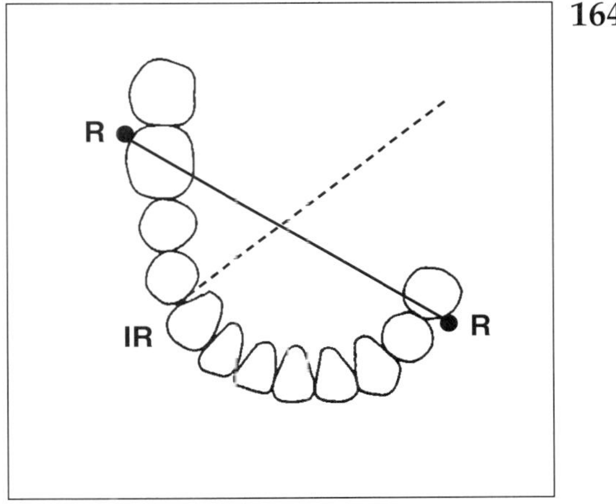

Fig **164** Retentive pattern.

Fig **165** Lingual extension of rest on to 47.
46 has a crown contoured for optimal shape.

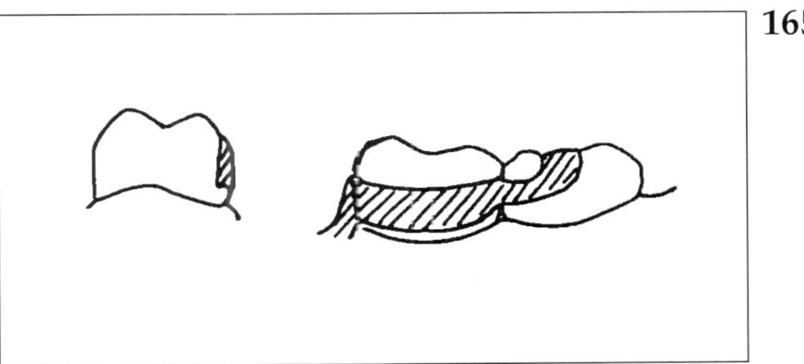

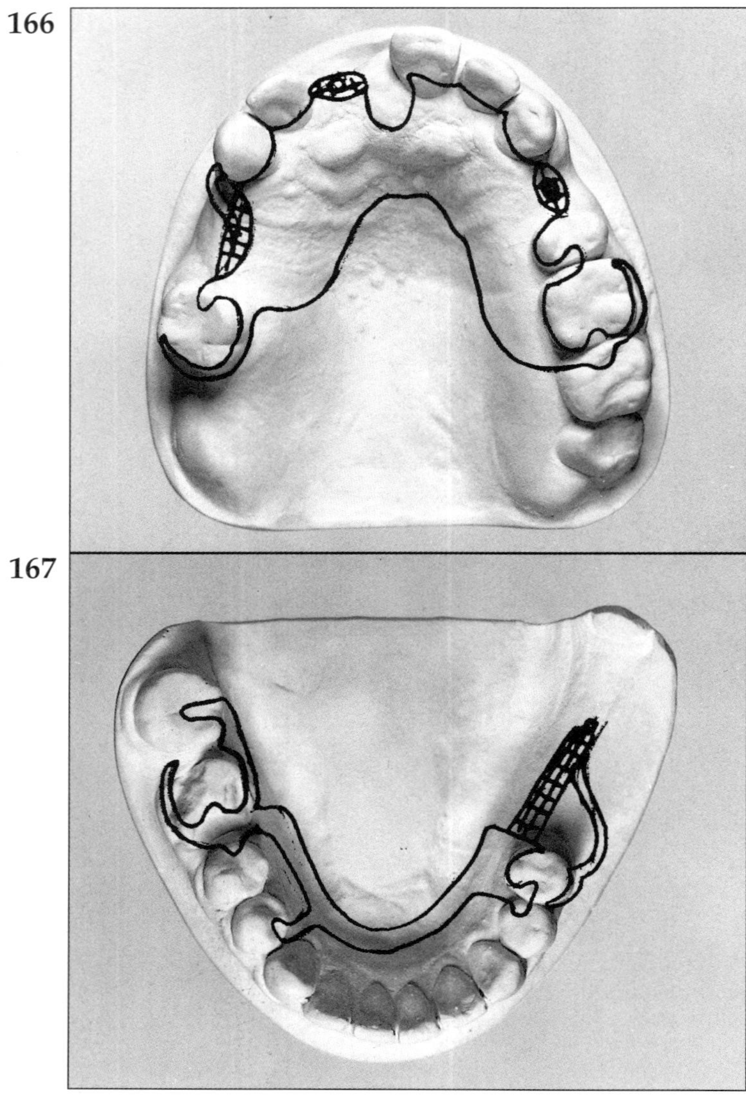

166

167

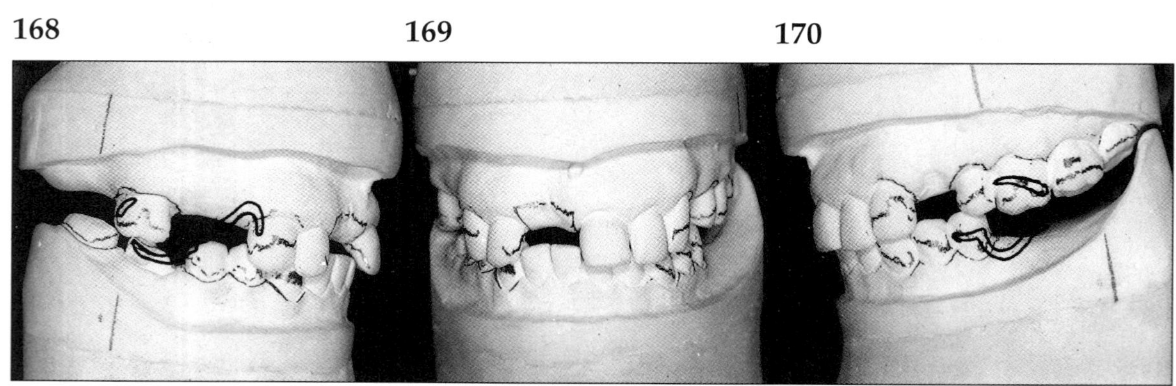

168 169 170

Patient No 4 (Figs 171–188)

History and examination

Name: R.N.N.

Sex: male

Age: 28 years

Occupation: factory foreman

c/o: acrylic partial upper denture broken

PDH: various upper dentures since age 18; fairly regular dental treatment

PMH: none relevant

o/e: wears maxillary RPD night and day; mild palatal hyperaemia; good gingival health

Radiographs: none available

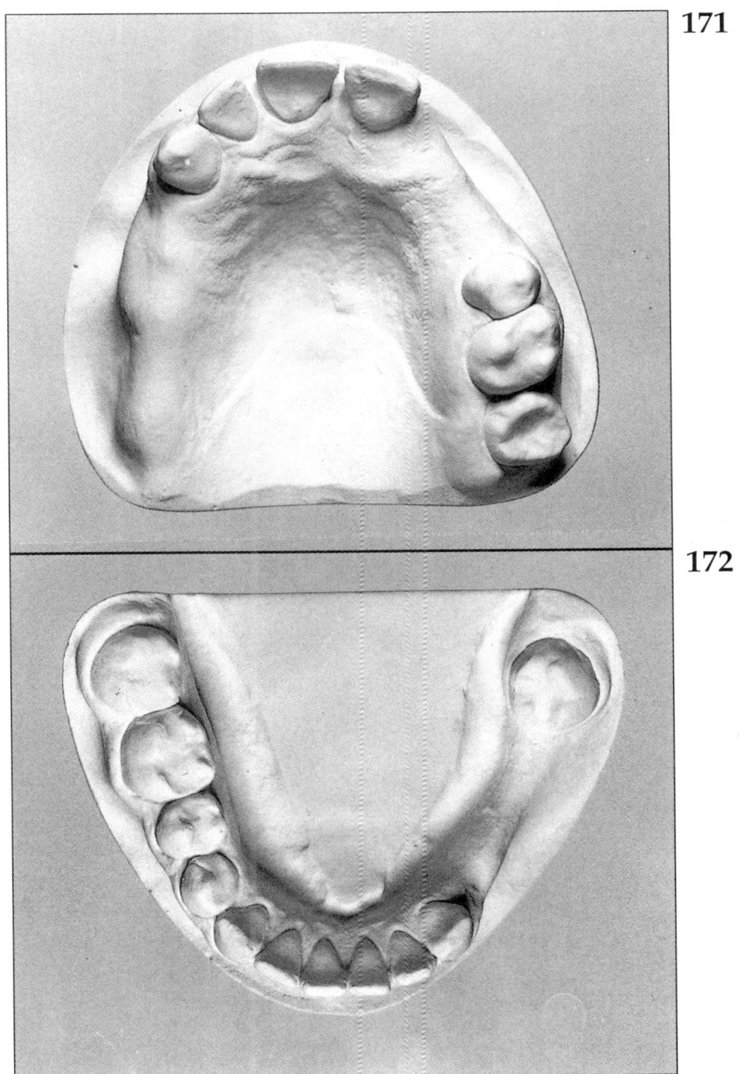

171

172

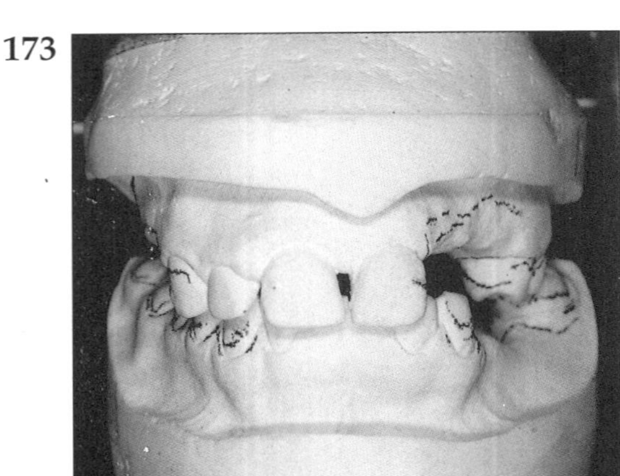

173

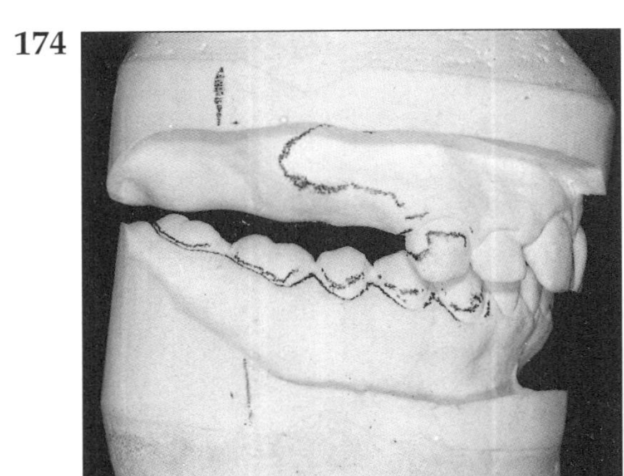

174

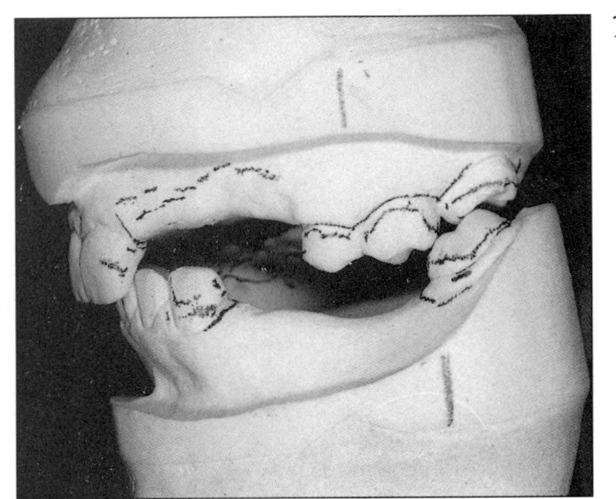

175

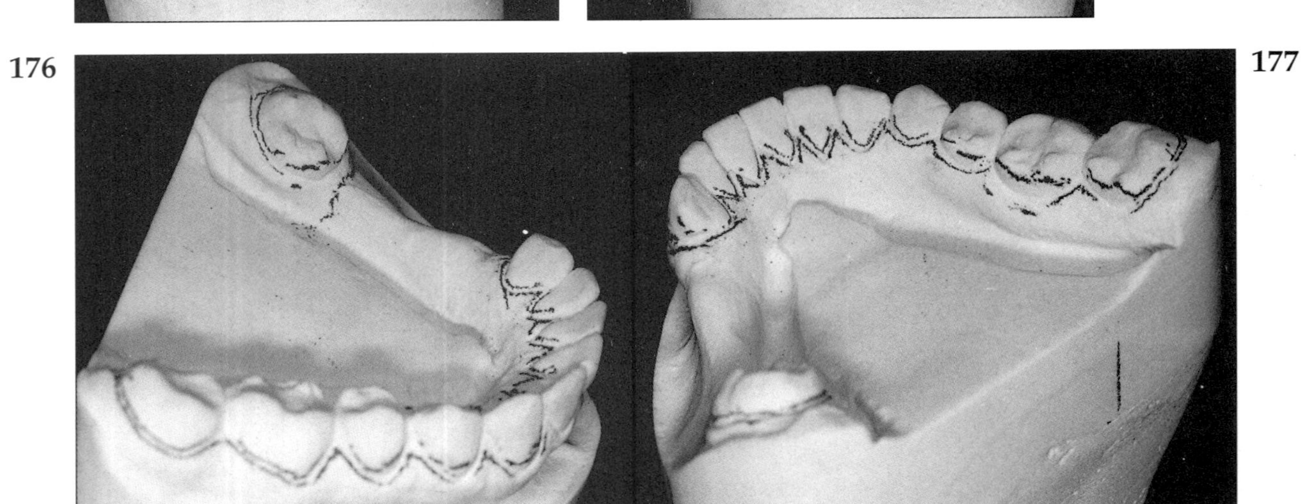

176

177

Treatment plan

Does this patient need RPD treatment?

The patient would like a maxillary prosthesis for aesthetics and for eating.

Dentally, both maxillary and mandibular prostheses would be desirable to prevent overeruption of 25 and 26 and of the lower right posteriors.

Treatment options

- Osseointegrated implants.
- RPD (acrylic or metal).

Decision and treatment plan

This is based on financial constraints:

- Complete restorative work and reduce overhanging margins (37).
- Counselling as regards leaving the denture out at night.
- Cobalt-chromium RPD.

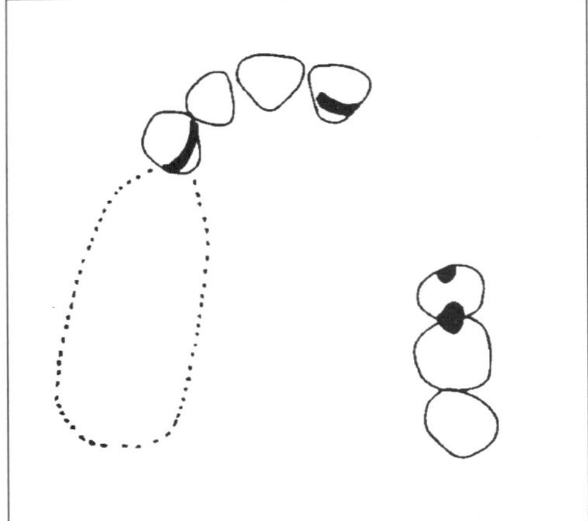

Fig **178** Support.

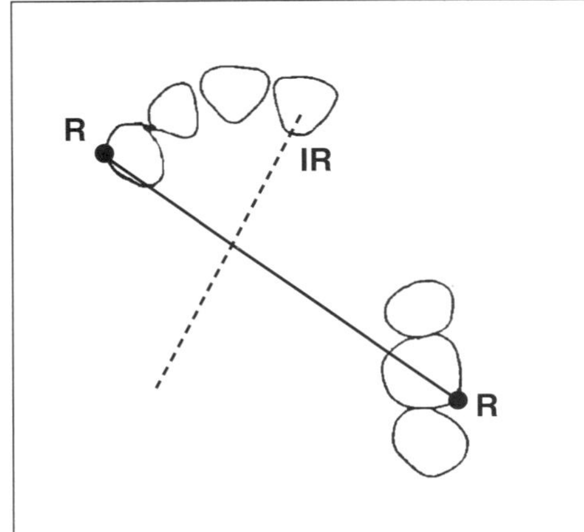

Fig **179** Retentive pattern.

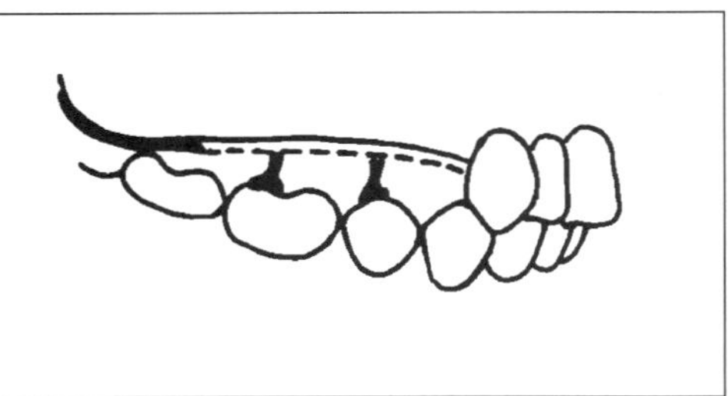

Fig **180** Metal studs provide occlusal stops.

Designs

Maxilla

Edentulous areas to be restored
1 tooth supported.
1 tooth and mucosa supported.

Support
- Occlusal rests 25(M) and (D) and 26(M).
- Cingulum rests 13 and 21.
- Maximum coverage of DE area.

Retentive pattern
Straight line between 13 and 26 augmented by guide planes on the proximal aspects of all abutments, and indirect retention on 21.

Retentive units
- 26 circumferential into DB (reciprocated by a palatal arm).
- 13 I-bar into DB (reciprocated by a palatal plate finishing on the MP surface).

Stabilisation
Palatal plate extending on to the MP surface of 13 prevents distal movement of the saddle.

Connector
Mid-palatal plate with polished surface extending over right tuberosity (page 35).

Acrylic anchorage
Grid for both edentulous areas with post for 22 and metal studs to provide occlusal stops against 45 and 46 (page 34).

Tooth modification
- Smooth occlusal rest areas.
- Guide planes on all proximal abutment surfaces and 13(MP).

Comments
- Occlusal rests on 25 and 26 will help to prevent overeruption of these teeth if the lower denture is not worn.
- A 'horseshoe' connector would give more mucosal support, but would be unaesthetic due to the diastemas. It would also cover the gingival margins.

Mandible

Edentulous areas to be restored
1 tooth supported.

Support
- Occlusal rest 37(ML).
- Cingulum rest 33.
- Additional occlusal rests 45(D) and 46(M) for cross-arch stabilisation.

Retentive pattern
Triangle between 37, 33 and 46 augmented by guide planes on 37 and 33.

Retentive units
- 37 short ring clasp into DL undercut (self-reciprocating).
- 33 I-bar into DB undercut (reciprocated by cingulum rest).
- 46 circumferential into DL undercut (reciprocated by a buccal arm).

Connector
Lingual plate changing to lingual bar beside 44 and 45 where space permits.

Stabilisation
See above (occlusal rests).

Acrylic anchorage
Mesh over edentulous area.

Tooth modification
- Smooth areas for occlusal rests.
- Lower survey line 37(MB).
- Guide planes on 37(M) and 33(D).

Comments
The ring clasp on 37 makes efficient use of the existing survey line. The MB undercut is too small for an inverted C-clasp.

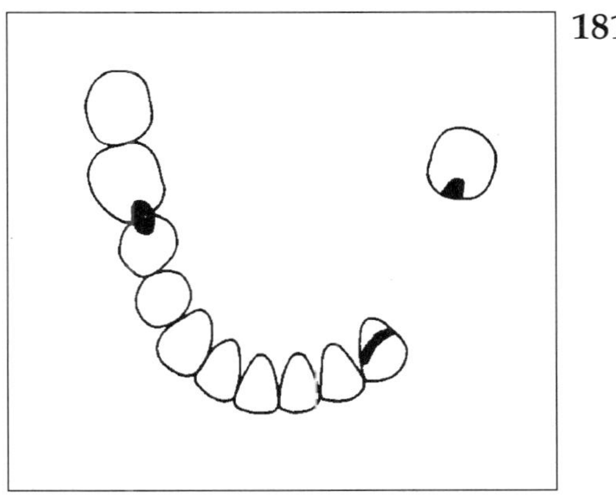

Fig **181** Support.

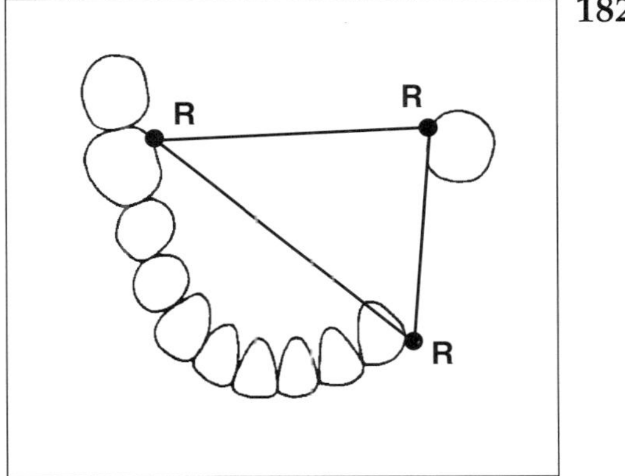

Fig **182** Retentive pattern.

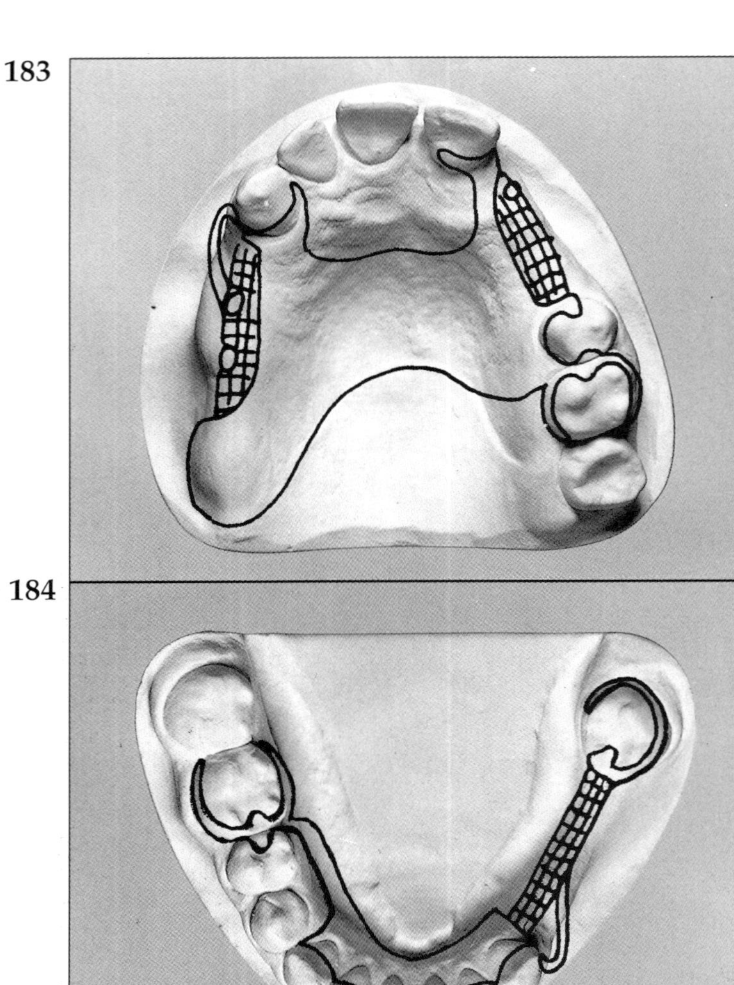

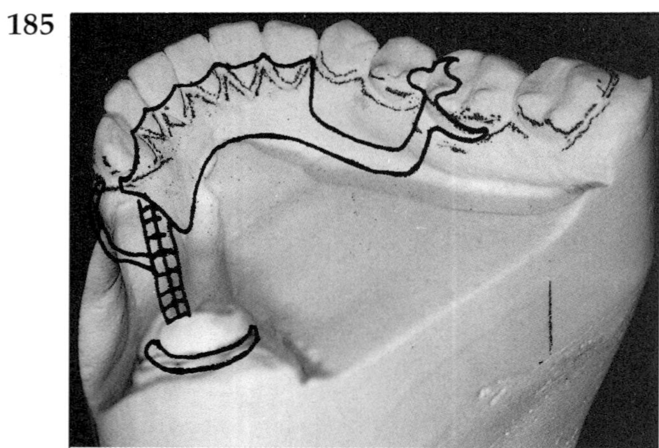

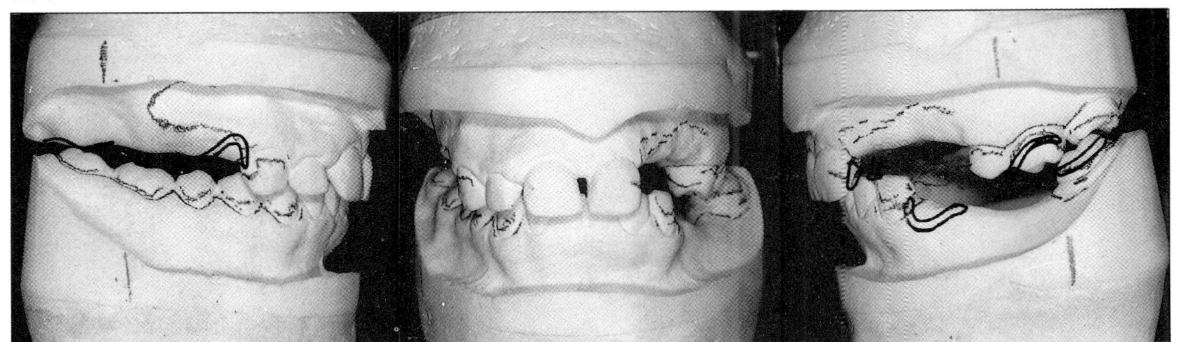

Patient No 5 (Figs 189–197)

History and examination

Name: B.R.M.　　　　　　*Sex:* female

Age: 30 years　　　　　　*Occupation:* housewife

c/o: wearing away front teeth; tooth broken upper left

PDH: regular attendance; recent history of grinding teeth; 25 restored composite a few months ago; eats both sides of mouth.

PMH: none relevant

o/e: no denture experience; right mandibular molars extracted late teens; good hygiene; 25 vital; enamel loss anterior maxillary teeth, especially 11 and 21

Radiographs: full mouth intra-oral

189

190

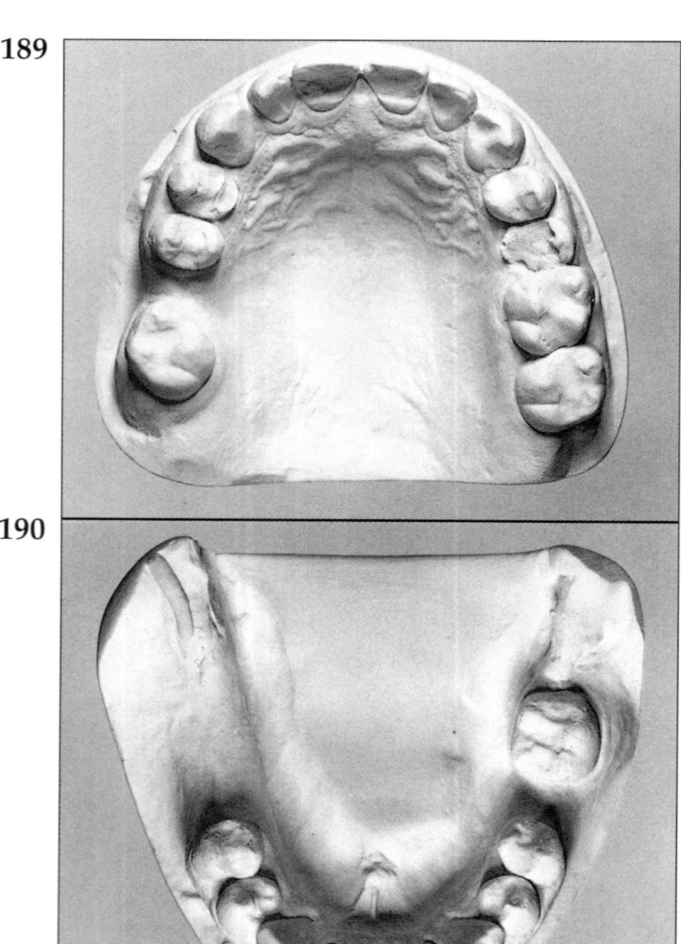

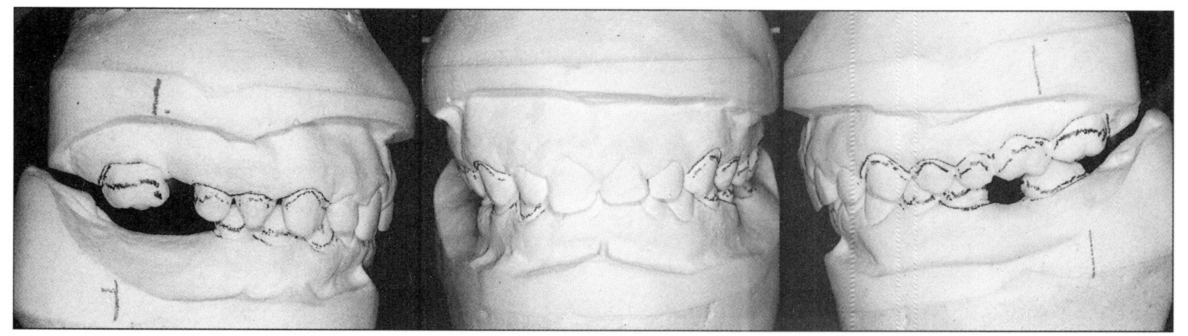

191   192   193

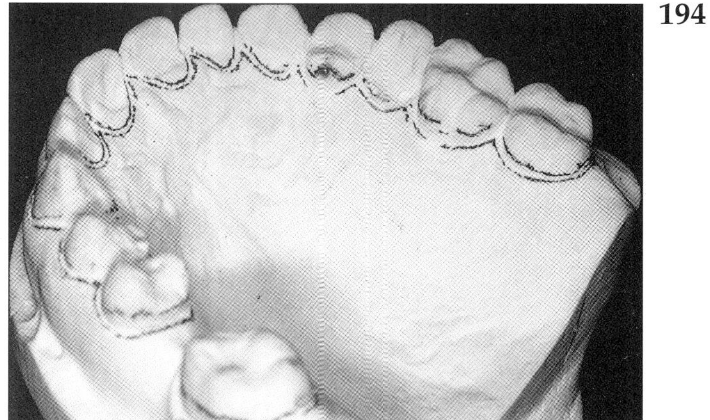

194

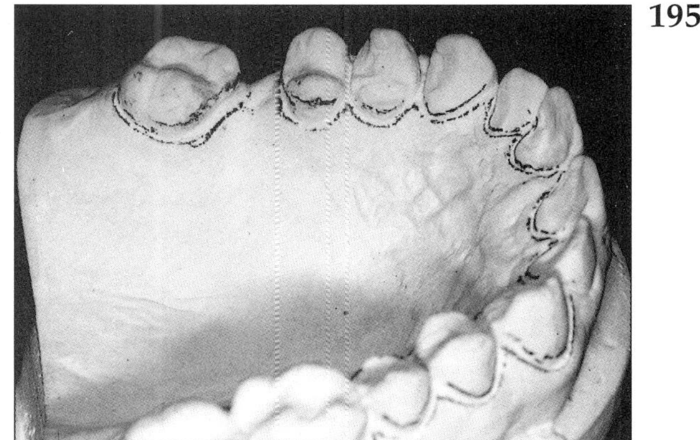

195

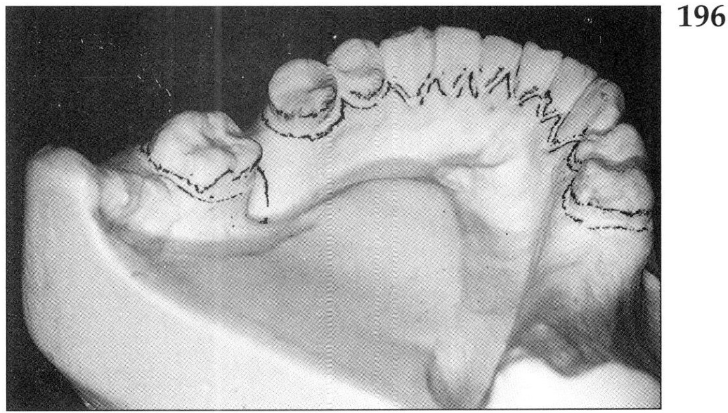

196

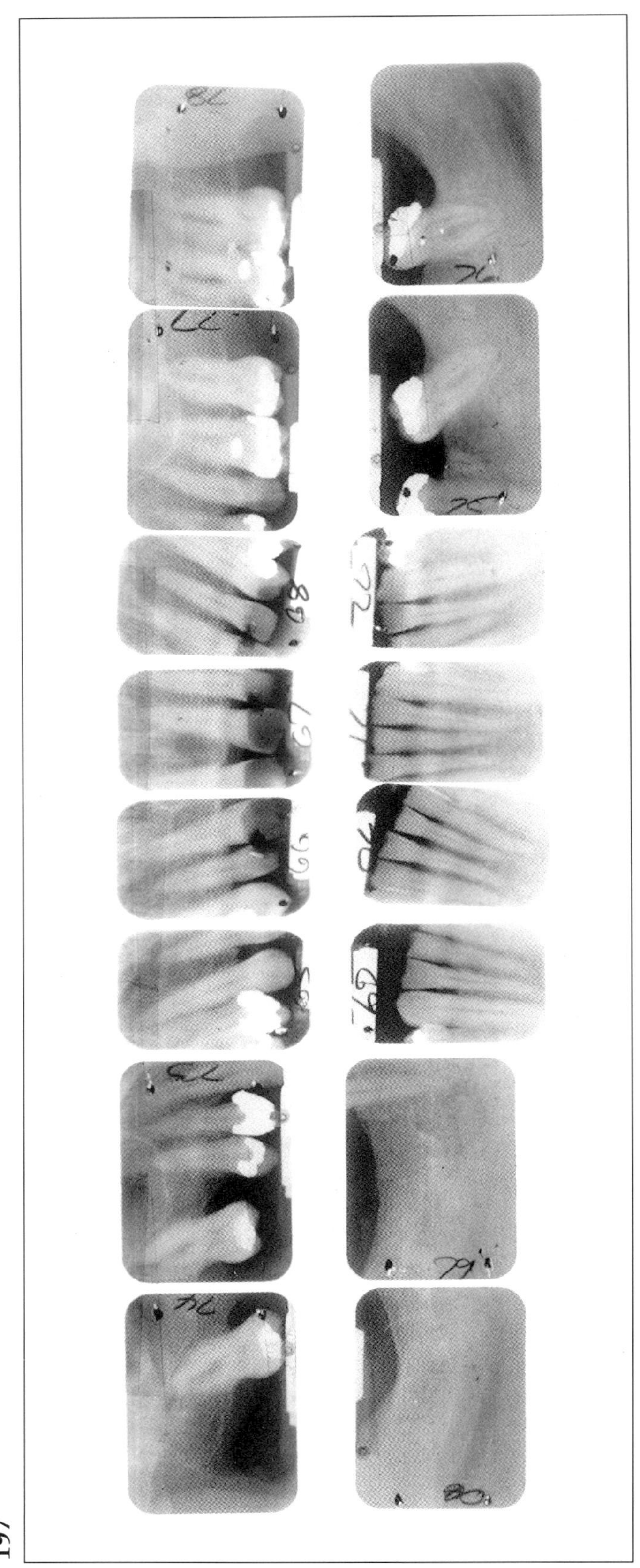

197

Treatment plan

Does this patient need RPD treatment?

The patient is concerned about her broken 25 and about her teeth 'wearing away'.

Dentally, there is danger of 17 overerupting, and of 15 and 27 moving distally and overerupting. Considerable wear on 11 and 21 could cause pulpal damage; 36 is unlikely to cause problems as it is locked in a stable position.

Treatment options

- Increase OVD with restorations.
- Fixed prosthesis 15–17 to stabilise the arch or extract 17 if problems occur.
- Osseointegrated implants in the lower right saddle.
- RPD (acrylic or metal) at increased OVD.

Decision

This is influenced by the probability that this patient is unlikely to wear removable dentures (there is no perceived benefit and the DEB will be uncomfortable) and by financial constraints precluding implants.

Treatment plan A

- Discuss the possible origins of (recent) tooth wear. Acrylic occlusal splint for maxilla (Michigan design), increasing OVD by not more than 1.5 mm. Monitor the patient's ability to cope with this increase in OVD.
- Serial replacement of maxillary restorations with metal (gold or amalgam) at new OVD. Adjust splint to accommodate restorations.
- Fixed restoration replacing 16 to stabilise the arch in this area.
- Restoration of palatal of upper anteriors with metal (gold or amalgam) providing occlusal stops.
- Restoration of the incisal shape and form 21.
- New acrylic splint to be worn at night and replaced as it wears out.

What should *not* be attempted is a combination of RPD, FPD and restorations where the occlusion becomes unstable if one or both RPD are not worn (page 13).

Treatment plan B

A maxillary overlay prosthesis, made in gold alloy, is an alternative if protection of maxillary incisors and premolars is considered essential. This would cover all maxillary teeth with a minimum thickness determined by the experience of the acrylic occlusal splint. The design of the occlusal surface of the removable overlay is the critical factor in success or failure, and a functionally generated path technique is advisable. This wax surface is made on an adjustable articulator in the first instance and then refined in the mouth before casting in yellow gold.

Patient No 6 (Figs 198–212)

History and examination

Name: I.B.　　　　　　　　　　*Sex:* female

Age: 48 years　　　　　　　　　*Occupation:* car sales

c/o: some difficulty in eating; feeling of tooth wear

PDH: fairly regular dental attendance; restoration of missing teeth was discussed in the past but was considered too expensive; no RPD experience

PMH: mild bronchitis, possibly connected with history of smoking

o/e: good hygiene; low caries status; occlusal restorations

Radiographs: full mouth intra-oral

198

199

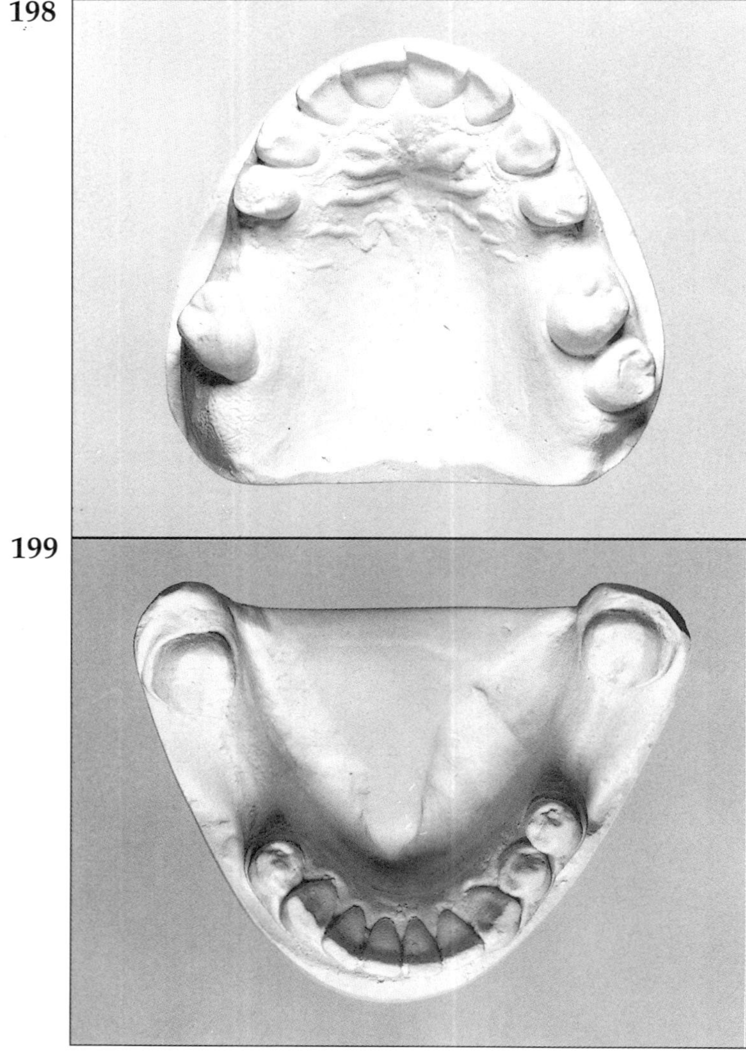

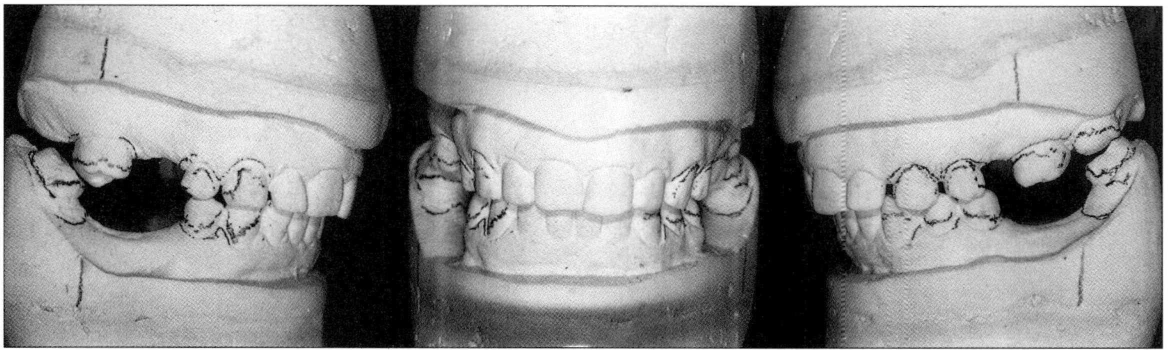

Treatment plan

Does this patient need RPD treatment?

The patient would like a prosthesis to make eating easier.

Dentally, the occlusal contact between 17 and 48 is unstable and likely to cause occlusal problems; 27 is less likely to cause damage since the opposing teeth have been lost for some time and overeruption is not evident.

Treatment options

- Fixed prostheses for all edentulous areas.
- RPD (acrylic or metal).

Decision

This is influenced by minimum finances and the patient's lack of perceived aesthetic problems.

- Lower cobalt-chromium RPD to give increased occlusal contacts for better mastication.
- Maxillary acrylic occlusal splint to be worn at night to lessen abrasion on maxillary incisors. This splint will be replaced as it wears out.

Note: an upper RPD would be more harmful than beneficial for this patient.

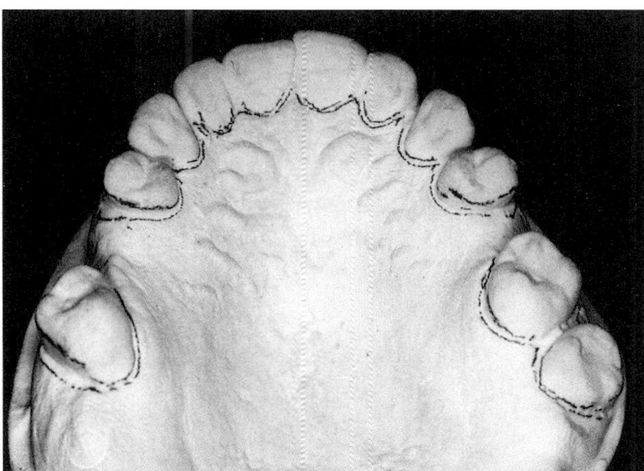

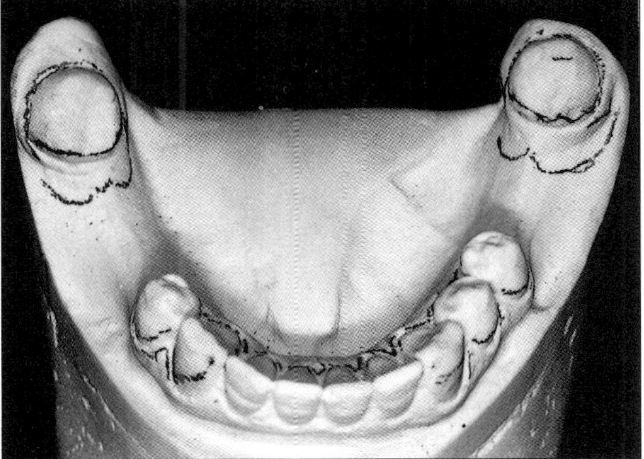

205

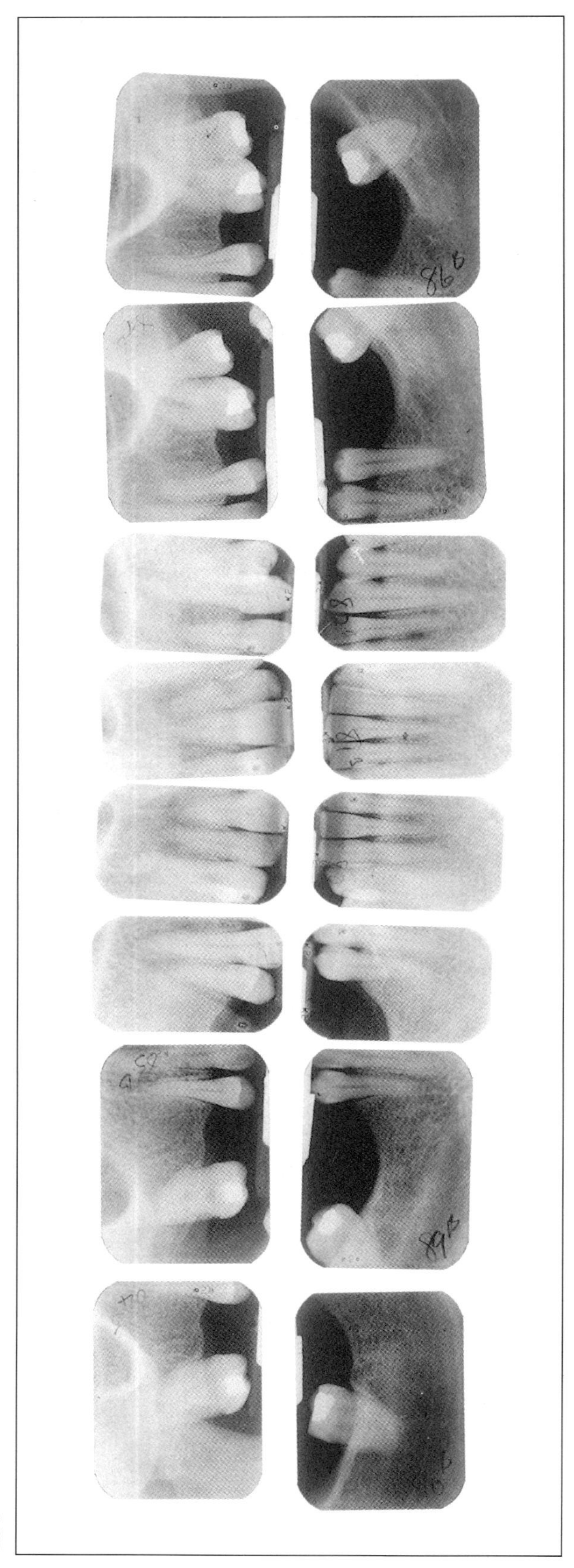

Design

Mandible

Edentulous areas to be restored
2 tooth supported

Support
Occlusal rests 38(M), 35(D), 44(D) and 48(MB) and (D).

Retentive pattern
Straight line between 35 and 48 augmented by guide planes and occlusal rests on 38 and 44 which prevent rotation.

Retentive units
- 48 ring clasp into ML undercut (self-reciprocating).
- 35 circumferential into MB undercut (reciprocated by lingual arm).

Connector
Lingual bar (or sublingual bar).

Tooth modification
- Occlusal adjustment as necessary to eliminate any slide caused by 17 and 48.
- Reduction of palatal cusps 17 to leave point contact between distal of 17 and occlusal 48.
- Smooth areas for occlusal rests.
- Lower survey line 48(MB).

Comments
A triangular retentive pattern would have been better than the straight line, but lack of suitable existing undercuts on 44 or 38 would make the design more complex; 48 has a D occlusal rest to help stabilise it.

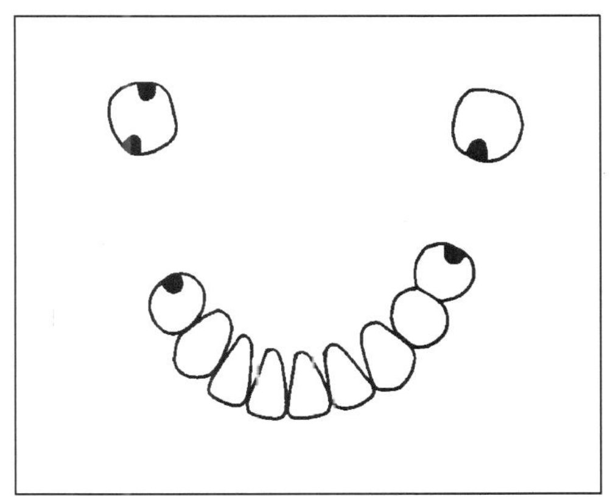

Fig **206** Support.

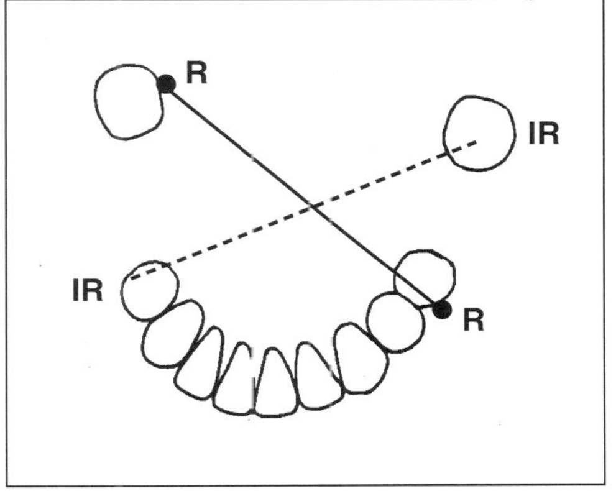

Fig **207** Retentive pattern.

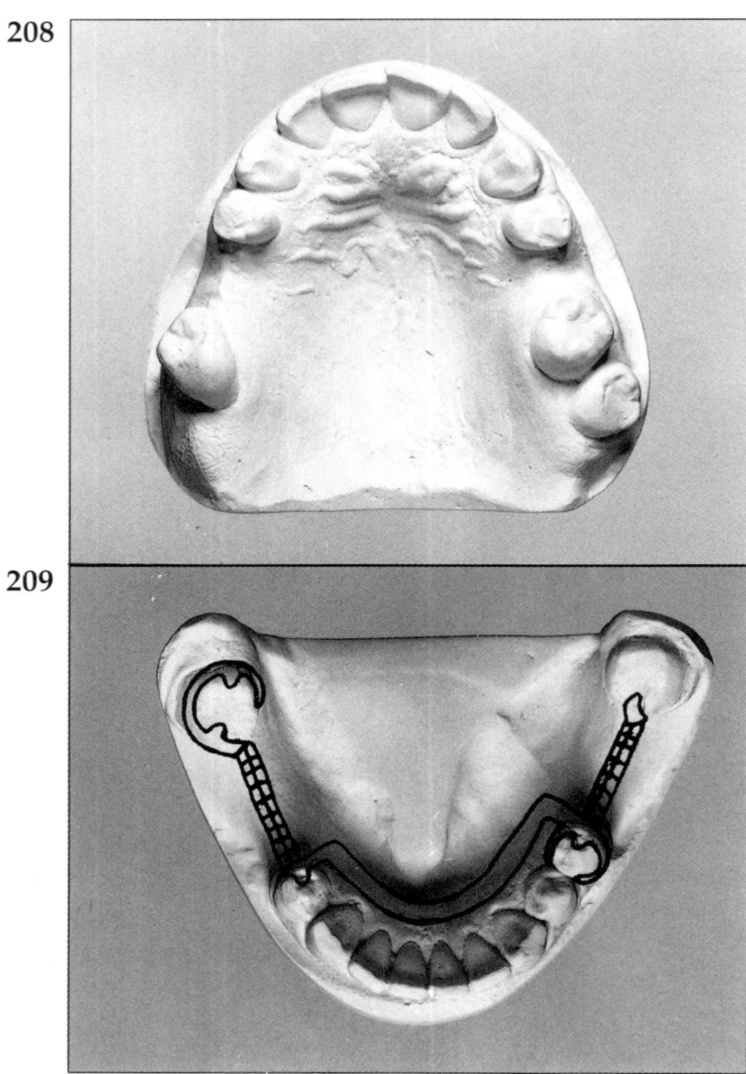

208

209

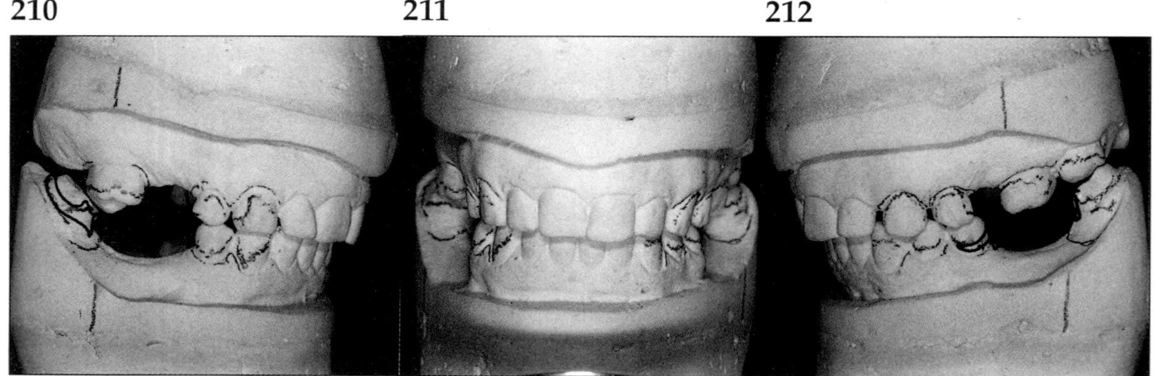

210   211   212

Patient No 7 (Figs 213–238)

History and examination

Name: D.R.H. *Sex:* male

Age: 53 years *Occupation:* physician

c/o: present acrylic RPD loose; some difficulty in eating

PDH: infrequent dental attendance; maxillary RPD is 6 years old with anterior palatal coverage, replacing 12 and 21 only; no experience of mandibular RPD

PMH: none relevant

o/e : marginal gingivitis in region of RPD; general standard of restorations good; oral hygiene average

Radiographs: full mouth intra-oral

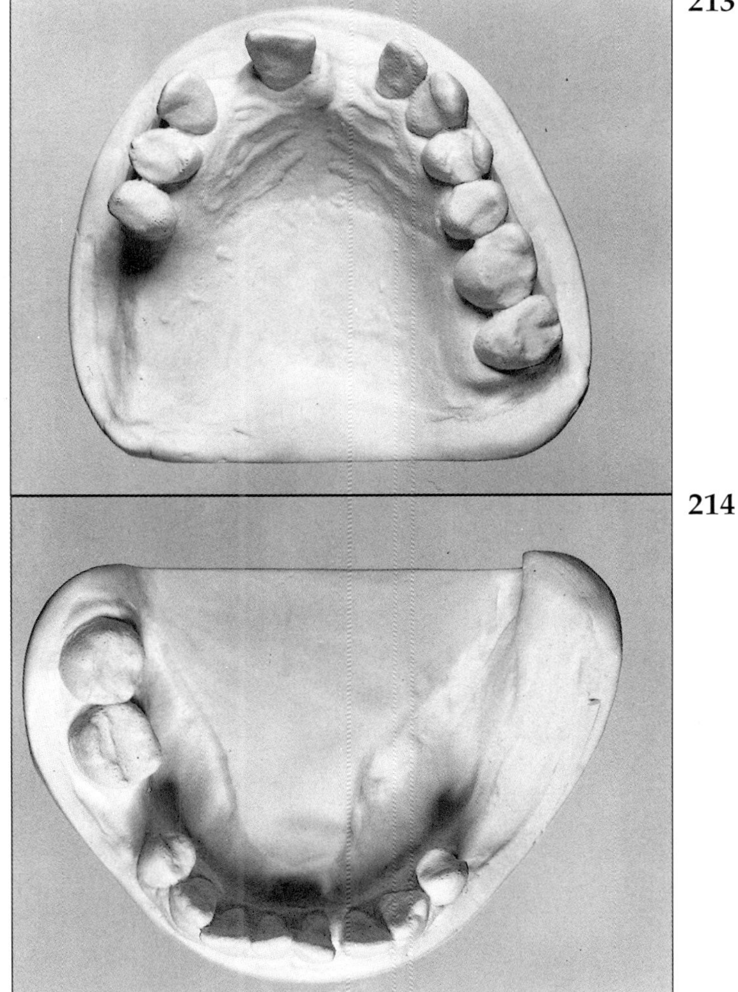

213

214

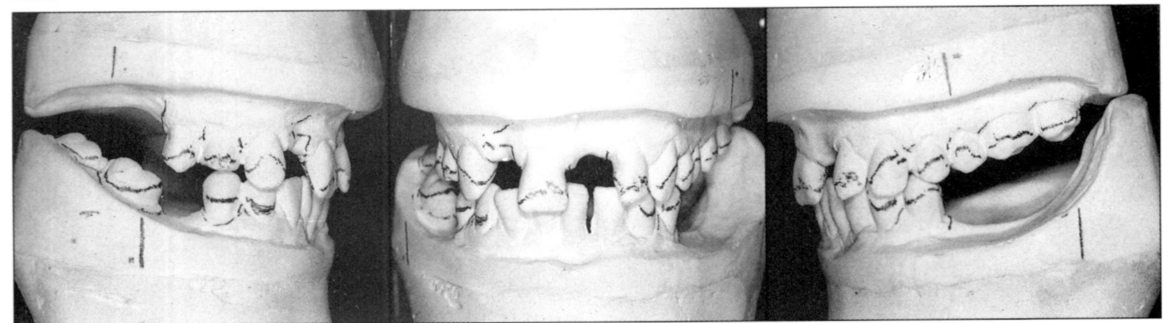

215   216   217

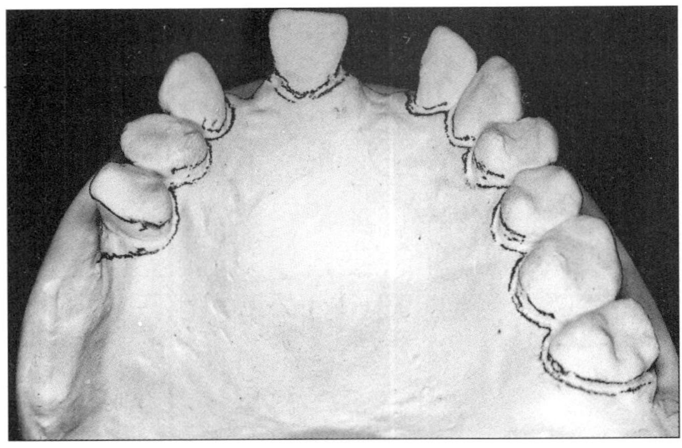

218

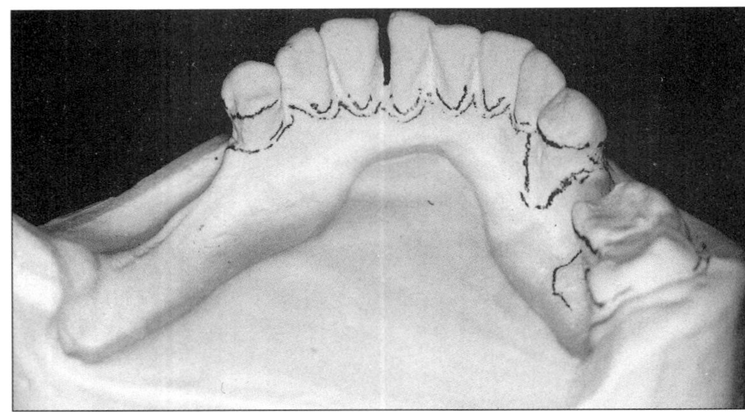

219

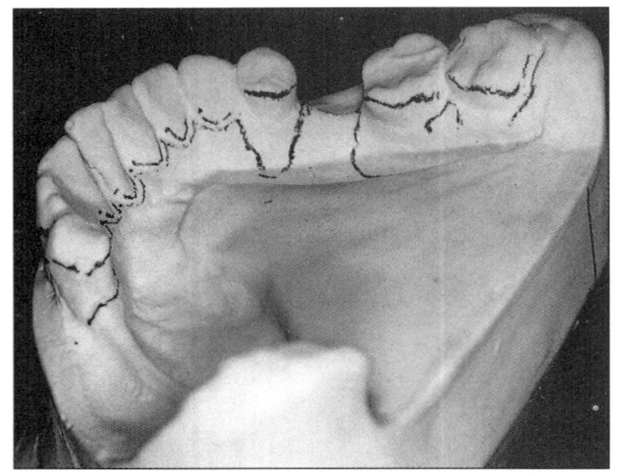

220

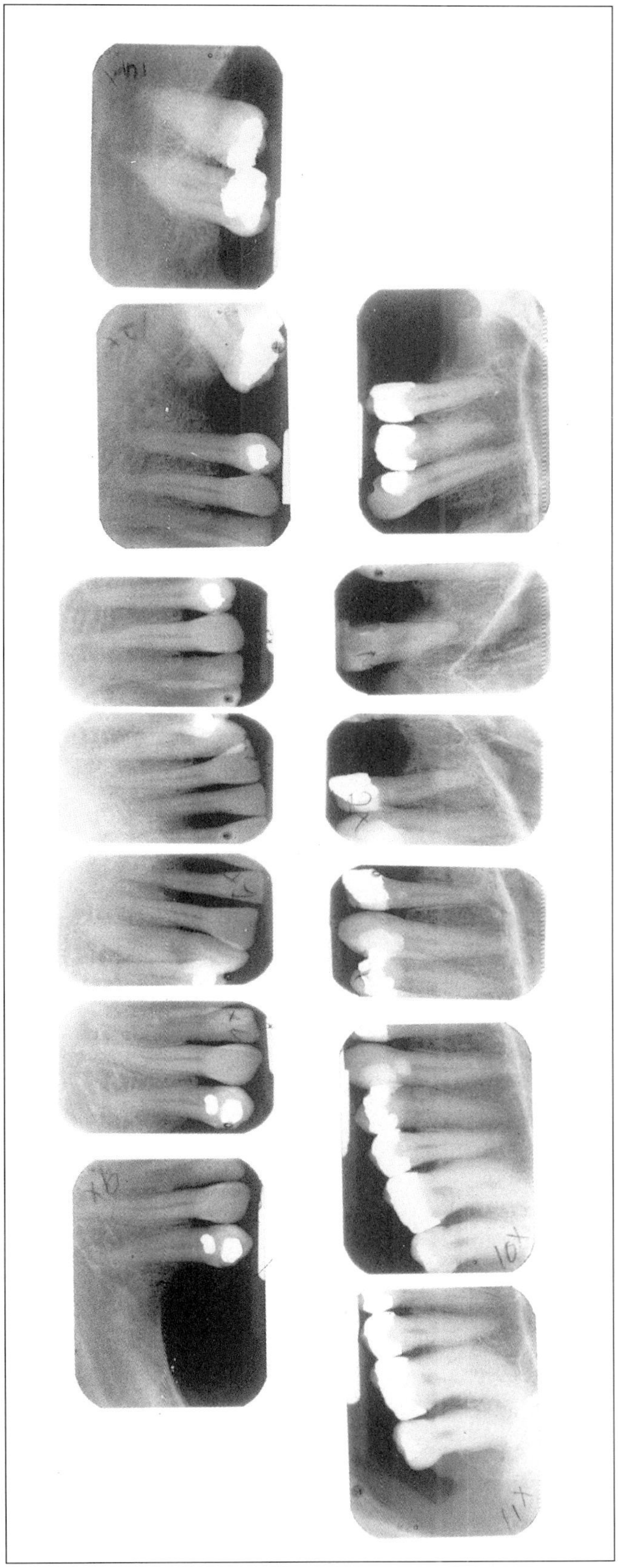

Treatment plan

Does this patient need RPD treatment?

The patient would like restoration of the anterior edentulous areas for aesthetics and at least one mandibular saddle for mastication.

Dentally, the left arch needs posterior support; 25, 26 and 27 are unlikely to overerupt (see patient's age); 46 and 47 have tilted and overerupted and need stabilisation.

Treatment options

MAXILLA
- Restore anterior edentulous areas only (fixed or removable).
- Extract 11 and 22 and make a fixed bridge.
- Restore the anterior and posterior edentulous areas (RPD metal or acrylic), with or without extraction of doubtful teeth.
- Osseointegrated implants.

MANDIBLE
- Nothing (if 46 and 47 are stabilised by an upper appliance).
- Fixed restoration right saddle.
- Osseointegrated implants.
- Metal RPD. A lower RPD should be avoided for this patient unless a sublingual bar is possible. Lack of space would preclude the use of a lingual bar. The periodontal condition contraindicates a lingual plate.

DECISION AND TREATMENT PLAN A (S.K.L.)
This is influenced by finances, space and available bone. The final decision as regards implants is based on data compiled from computer-assisted tomograms.

- Prophylaxis and oral hygiene instruction.
- Extraction 47 (overerupted), 27 (beyond possibility of stabilisation), 11 (poor prognosis).
- Temporary immediate upper RPD (see design A).
- Implants placed in upper anterior saddle and lower left saddle.
- Fixed conventional prosthesis replacing 45.
- Fixed restorations on implants.
- Strict recall and maintenance programme.

DECISION AND TREATMENT PLAN B (A.R.M.)
In spite of a reduced alveolar foundation and marginal gingivitis for a number of maxillary teeth, for example, 15, 11 and 22, the general periodontal condition is optimistic. Therefore, a decision is made to proceed to a replacement maxillary RPD.

The difficulties of unilateral DEB designs in mandibular RPDs present problems, but in order to produce a functional occlusion, a tooth and mucosa-borne denture is planned.

- Treatment of marginal gingivitis by tissue conditioner in the existing RPD and careful oral hygiene measures.
- Upper and lower cobalt-chromium RPD.
- Strict recall and maintenance programme.

Design A (S.K.L.)

Maxilla

Edentulous areas to be restored
1 tooth supported.

Support
- Occlusal rest 14(M).
- Rigid part of clasp between 25 and 26, and between 23 and 24.
- Cingulum 13 and 23.

Retentive pattern
Triangle between 15, 23 and 26.

Retentive units
- 15, circumferential from mid-palatal to DB surface.
- 23, short circumferential into DB undercut.
- 26, embrasure clasp across occlusal and into DB undercut.

Connector
Acrylic 'horseshoe' plate.

Tooth modification
Nil. This is a temporary appliance only. The final restoration will not involve the remaining maxillary teeth.

Comments
The base must be entirely tooth supported to allow relief on the tissue fitting surface while osseointegration takes place.

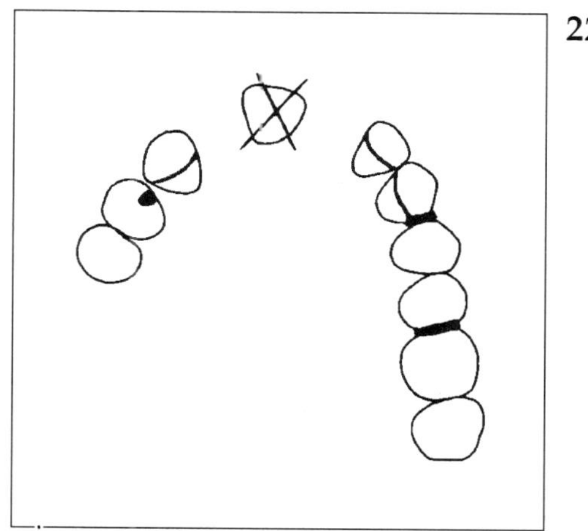

Fig **222** Support.

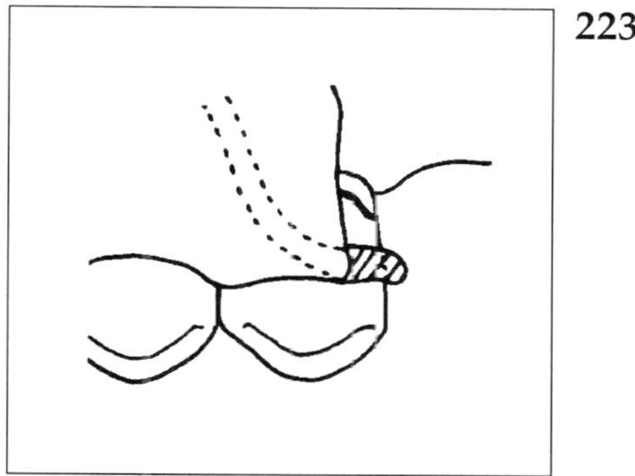

Fig **223**   Retainer on 15; palatal surface.

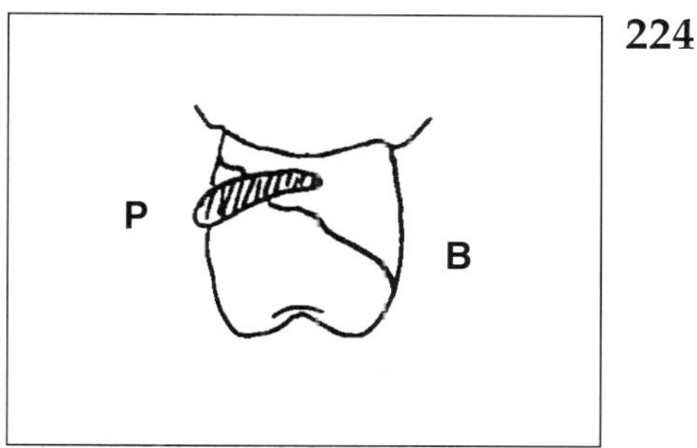

Fig **224** Retainer on 15; distal surface.

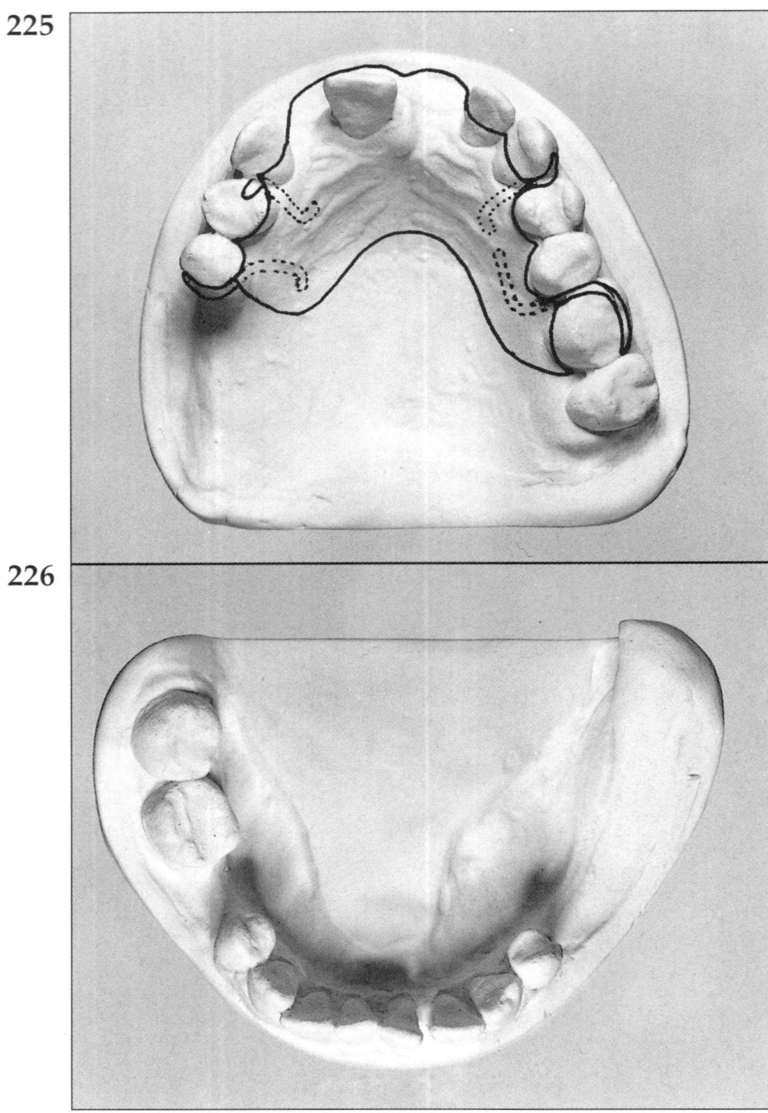

225

226

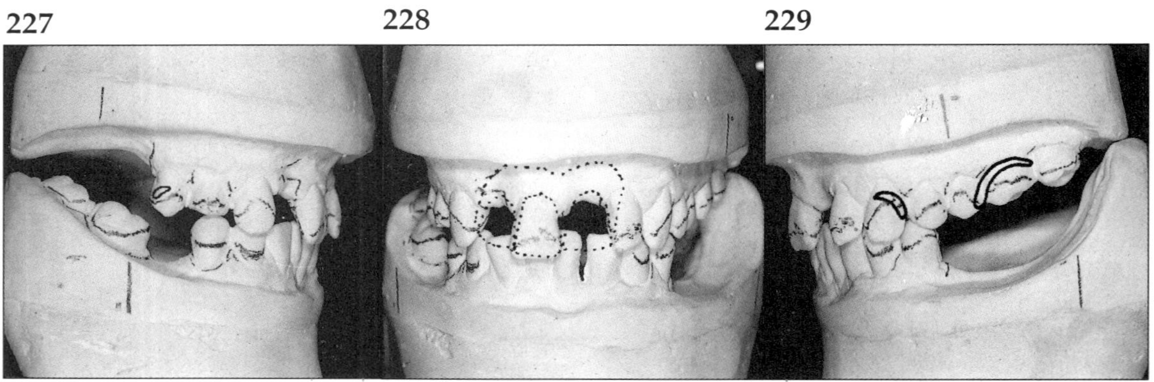

227 228 229

Design B (A.R.M.)

Maxilla

Sectional denture. The two parts are linked by two stainless steel (SS) tubes (internal diameter 1.3 mm) in the main component, and two SS pins (1.3 mm diameter) in the anterior component.

EDENTULOUS AREAS
2 tooth supported.
1 tooth and mucosa supported.

SUPPORT
- Occlusal rests 15(M), 14(D), 26(D) and 27(D).
- Cingulum rests 13 and 23.

RETENTIVE PATTERN
Triangle between 15 and 27, and anterior edentulous areas. Insertion of the anterior component is parallel to the occlusal plane; insertion of the main component is at right angles to the occlusal plane.

RETENTIVE UNITS
- 27 circumferential into MB undercut (reciprocated by plate).
- 15 L-bar into MB undercut (reciprocated by plate).

CONNECTION
Ring of sufficient dimension for cross-arch bracing.

ACRYLIC ANCHORAGE
- Anterior component comprises labial flange from right canine eminence to left lateral, denture teeth 12 and 21 and two patrix pins.
- Mesh over posterior edentulous area.

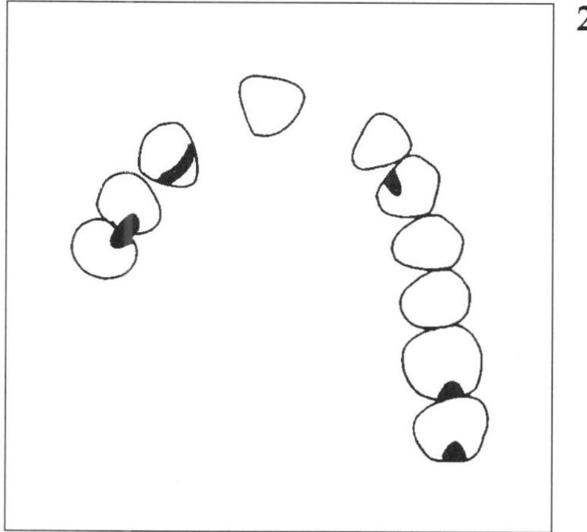

Fig **230** Support.

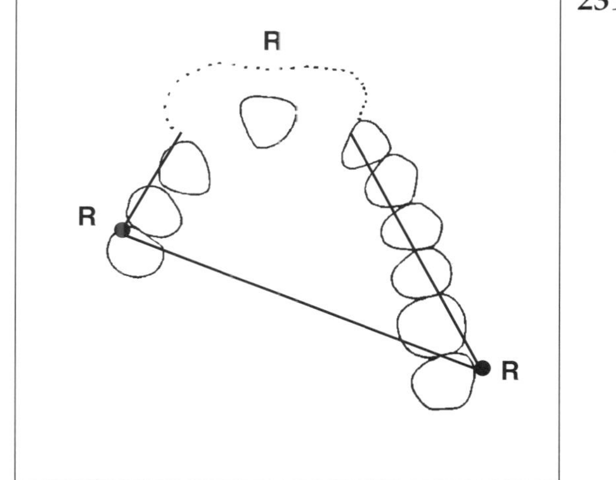

Fig **231** Retentive pattern.

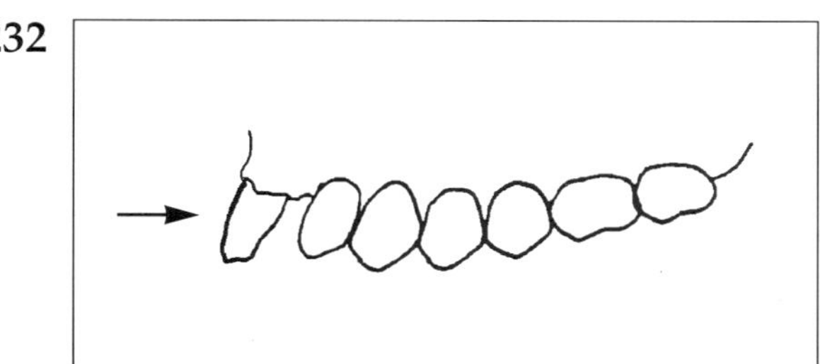

Fig **232** Insertion of anterior component.

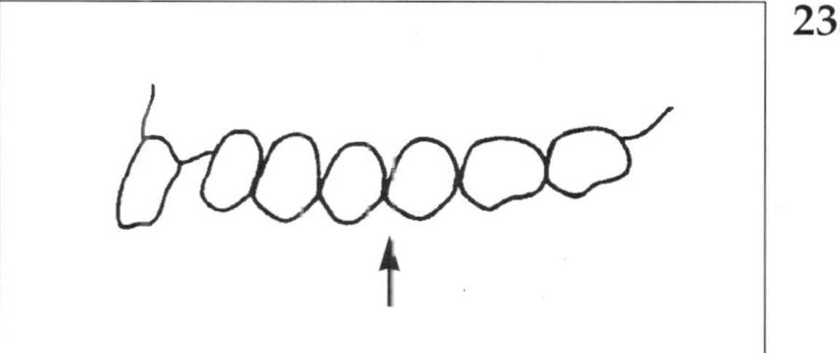

Fig **233** Insertion of posterior component.

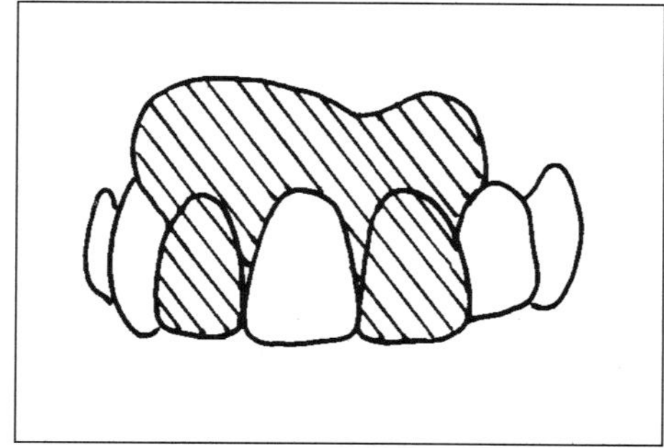

Fig **234** Anterior flange.

TOOTH MODIFICATION
- Rest seat preparation in six abutments.
- Discing mesial and distal surfaces of 13, 11 and 22 to ensure intimate fit of labial flange.

COMMENTS

The main component must be retentive by itself. The linking of the two components by pin and tube ensures a very positive resistance to displacement.

The wide labial flange, correctly contoured with the correct colour match, ensures excellent aesthetics provided the chamfered edge stops on unresorbed tissue. Oral hygiene must be carefully controlled.

Mandible

EDENTULOUS AREAS TO BE RESTORED
2 tooth supported.
1 tooth and mucosa supported.

Support:
- Occlusal rests 46(M), 44(D) and 34(M).
- Incisal rests 43(D) and 33(D).
- Mucosal support: wide extension and altered cast technique.

RETENTIVE PATTERN
Straight line between 34 and 44 augmented by indirect retainers extended on cingulum of 43 and 33.

RETENTIVE UNITS
- Circumferential 44 (reciprocated by lingual arm),
- I-bar 34 (reciprocated by lingual plate).

CONNECTOR
Sub-lingual bar ensuring adequate cross-arch bracing, necessary because of the long, atrophic distal extension area.

TOOTH MODIFICATION
- Guide planes 46(M), 44(D) and 34(D).
- Incisal rest seats 43(D) and 33(D).

COMMENTS
The 'at risk' abutment is 34, particularly because of the alveolar bone lost distal to it. Full veneer crowns on 33 and 34, joined to form a combined abutment, would be an advantage.

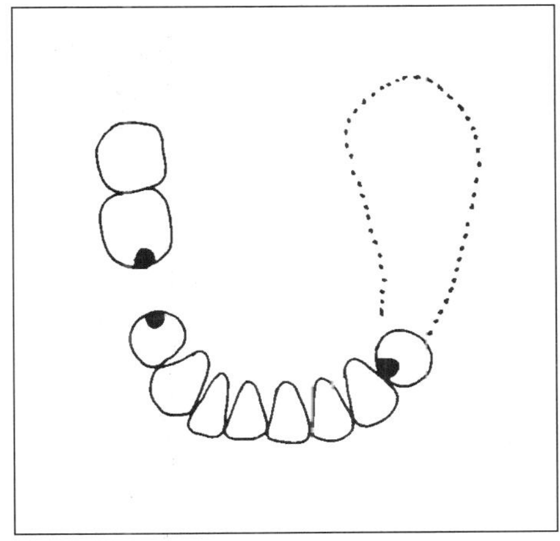

Fig **235** Support.

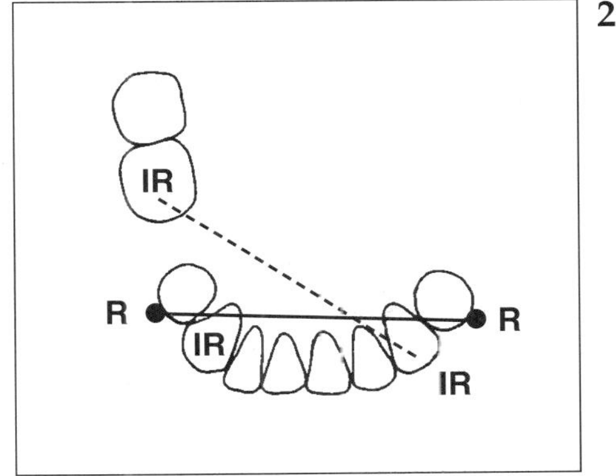

Fig **236** Retentive pattern.

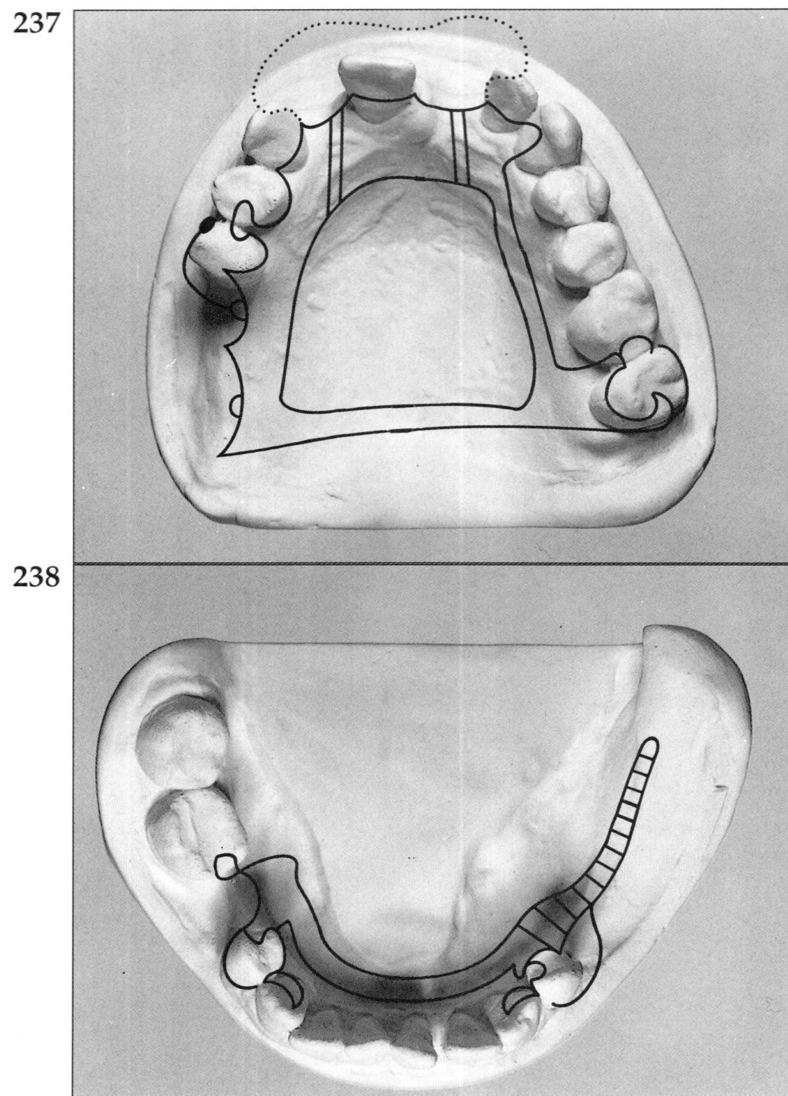

237

238

Patient No 8 (Figs 239–256)

History and examination

Name: A.Y.
Sex: male
Age: 41 years
Occupation: journalist
c/o: anterior teeth chipping; some difficulty in chewing
PDH: infrequent dental visits; upper acrylic partial denture about 4 years old but not always worn; lower partial denture made some time ago but never worn because it felt 'unpleasant'
PMH: none relevant
o/e: upper anteriors temporarily restored with composite; oral hygiene good, healthy gingivae
Radiographs: full mouth intra-oral

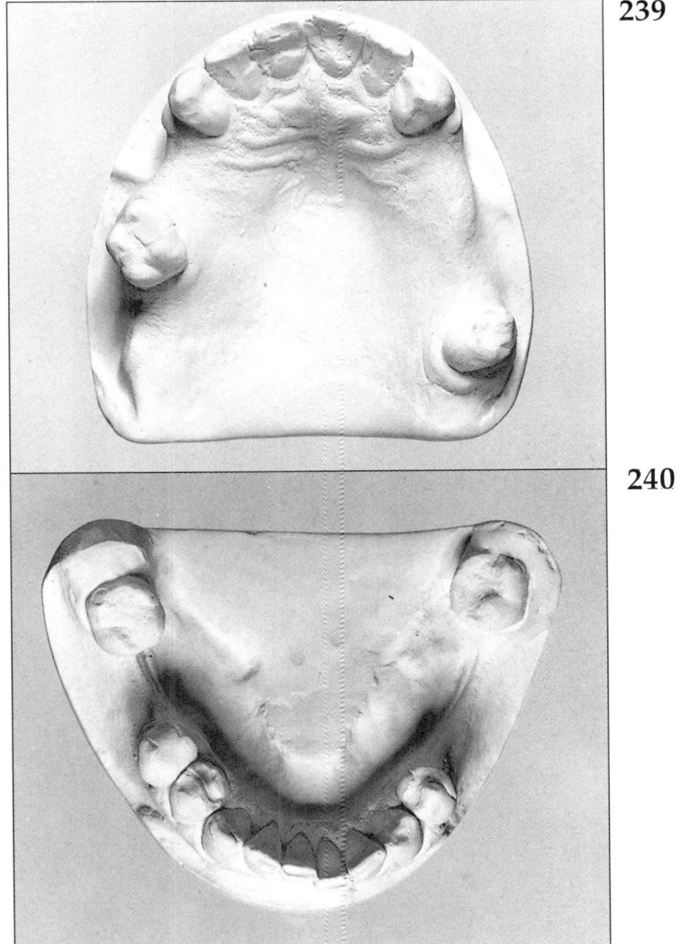

239

240

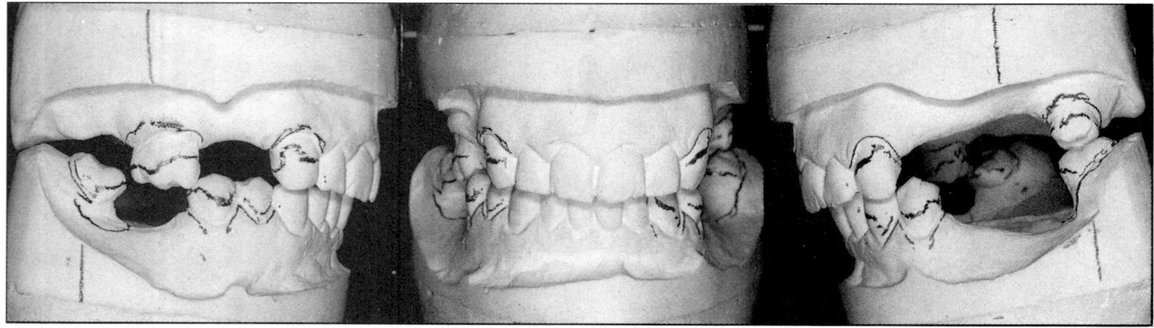

241 242 243

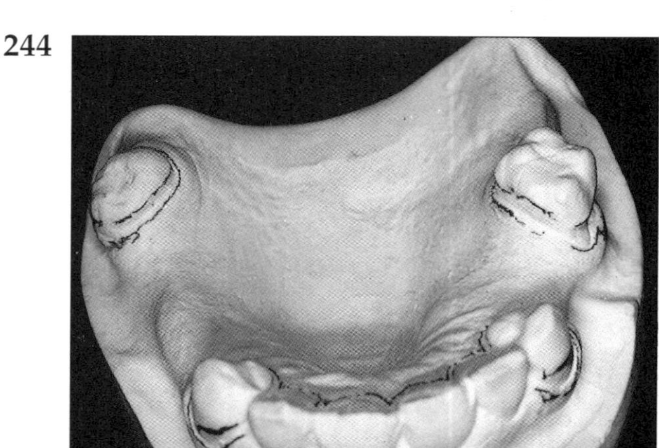

244

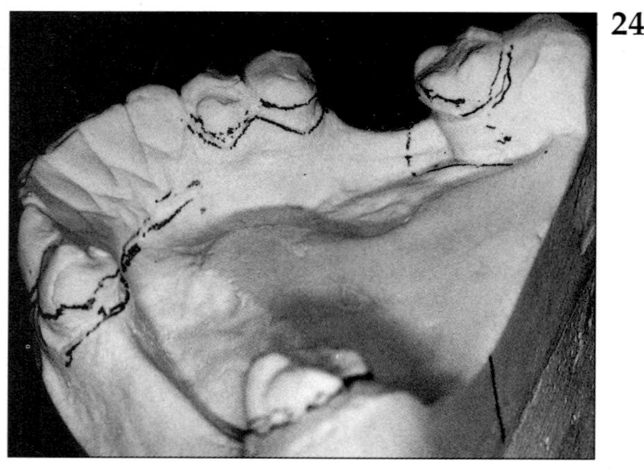

245

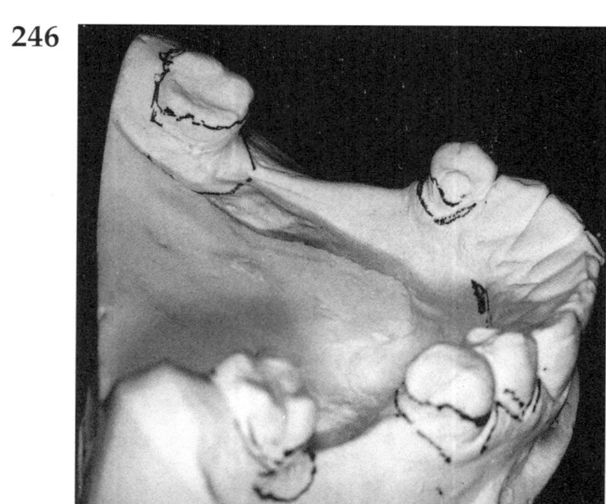

246

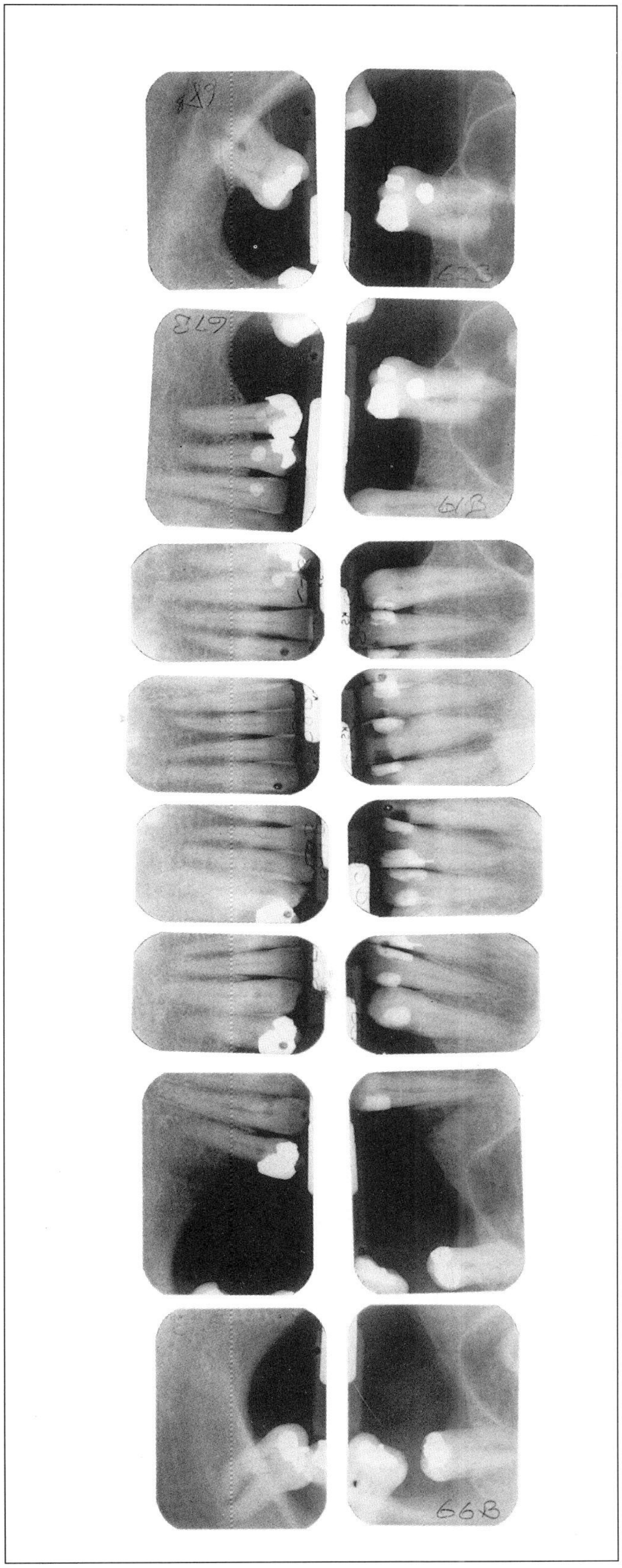

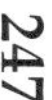

Treatment plan

Does this patient need RPD treatment?

The patient is worried about the anterior teeth chipping and lack of masticating surfaces.

Dentally, there is a lack of posterior occlusal stops and potential overeruption of 16 causing a locked occlusion.

Treatment options

Maxilla
- Restore anteriors as necessary.
- RPD (acrylic or metal).
- Osseointegrated implants.

(Fixed prostheses are contraindicated due to the length of the edentulous areas.)

Mandible
- RPD (acrylic or metal).
- Osseointegrated implants.

(Fixed prostheses are contraindicated due to the length of edentulous areas.)

Decision and treatment plan

This is influenced by finances and the patient's wishes after an explanation of the necessity for posterior occlusal support. The treatment plan must take into consideration that the patient may not wear the lower RPD.

- Examination of the old lower RPD to discover what was 'unpleasant'.
- Replace the restoration on 23(D) with amalgam or gold. Incorporate an undercut in this restoration.
- Upper and lower RPDs (cobalt-chromium).
- Replace restorations on maxillary anteriors. Restorations would normally be completed prior to the construction of dentures. In this case the dentures are needed to provide posterior support before the restorations are placed.
- Maxillary acrylic splint to be worn at night and replaced as it wears.

Designs

Maxilla

Edentulous areas
2 tooth supported.

Support
* Occlusal rests 16(MP) and 28(M).
* Cingulum rests 13 and 23.

Retentive pattern
Triangle between 16, 13 and 23, augmented by guide planes on all proximal surfaces and by indirect retention (OR on 28).

Retentive units
* 16 ring clasp into DB undercut (self-reciprocating).
* 13 and 23 I-bars into DB undercuts (reciprocated by cingulum rest).

Connector
Mid-palatal bar.

Acrylic anchorage
Mesh over saddle areas.

Tooth modification
* Smooth occlusal rest areas.
* Prepare cingulum rests.
* Guide planes on proximal of abutments.

Comments
The retentive triangle is small because 16 and 13 are close together. 16, 23 and 28 would have given a better retentive pattern but lack of viable undercuts on 28 have made this untenable.

The occlusal rest on 16 is on the MP surface since the mesial has occlusal contact with 45.

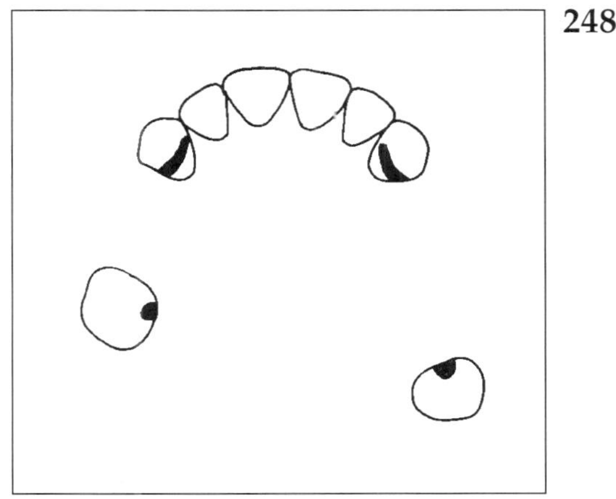

Fig **248** Support.

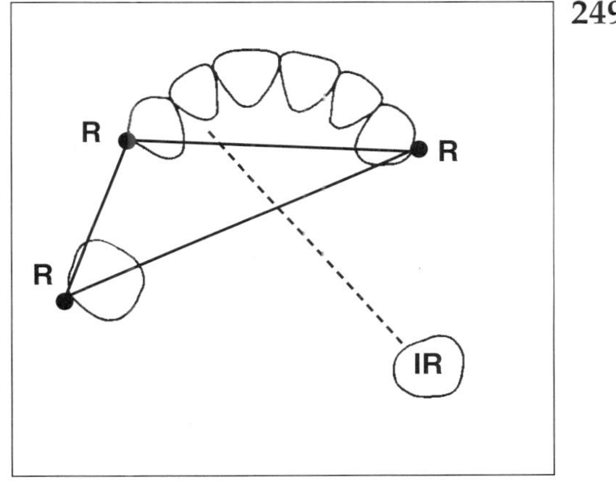

Fig **249** Retentive pattern (note that the triangle is too small for adequate retention without indirect retention).

"

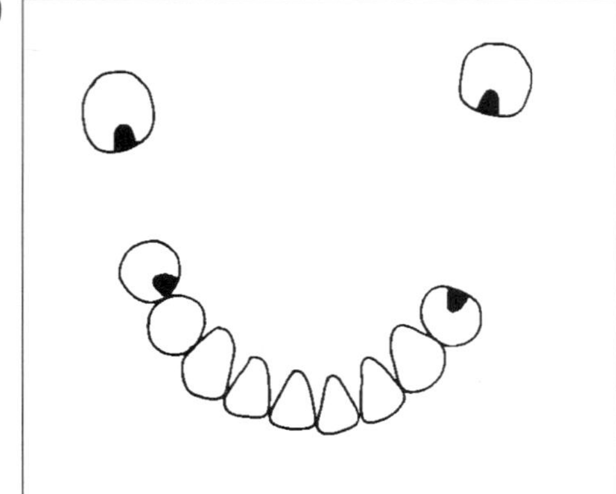

Fig **250** Support.

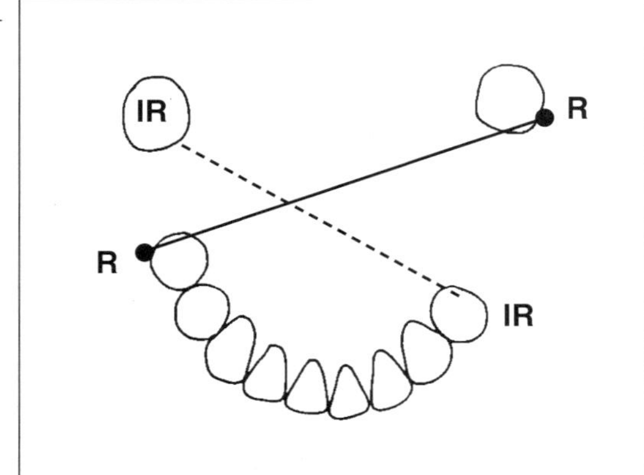

Fig **251** Retentive pattern.

Mandible

EDENTULOUS AREAS
2 tooth supported.

SUPPORT
Occlusal rests 37(M), 34(D), 45(M, since D has occlusal contact with 16) and 47(M).

RETENTIVE PATTERN
Straight line between 37 and 45 augmented by guide planes and occlusal rests on 34 and 47.

RETENTIVE UNITS
- 37 inverted C into MB undercut (reciprocated by lingual arm).
- 45 I-bar into DB undercut (reciprocated by lingual plate).

CONNECTOR
Lingual plate.

ACRYLIC ANCHORAGE
Mesh over saddle areas.

TOOTH MODIFICATION
- Smooth areas for occlusal rests.
- Lower survey line 37 lingual for rigid reciprocator.
- Guide planes on proximal surfaces.

COMMENTS
A lingual plate is used here as there is insufficient space for a lingual bar. A sublingual bar could have been used if anatomy permitted.

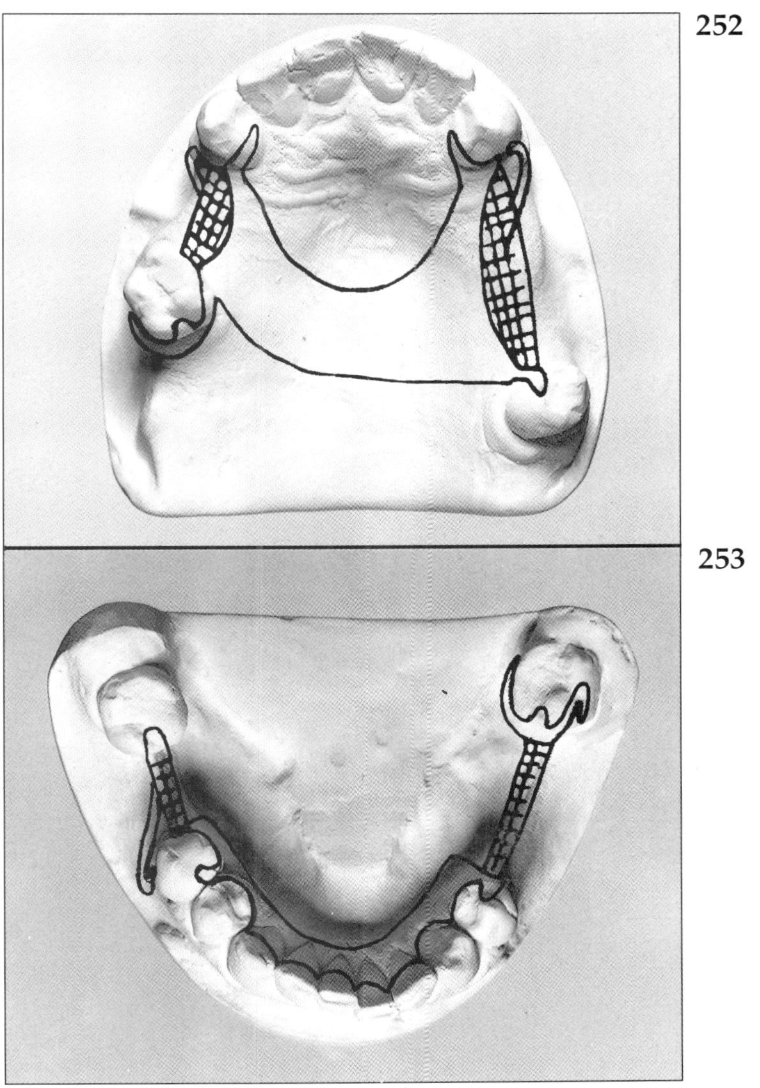

252

253

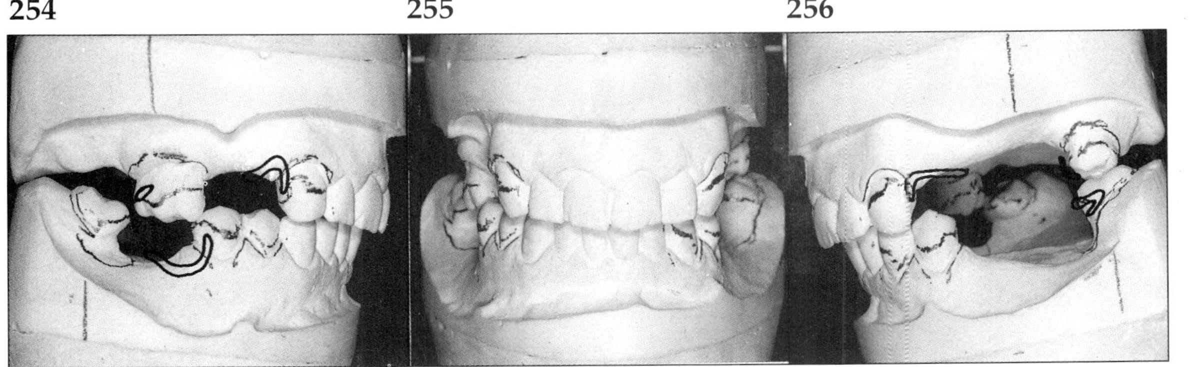

254   255   256

Patient No 9 (Figs 257–275)

History and examination

Name: N.T.　　　　　　　　　　*Sex:* female

Age: 47 years　　　　　　　　　*Occupation:* shopkeeper

c/o: metal partials made in last few months by another dentist who has now gone overseas; neither denture feels comfortable

PDH: received upper and lower RPD to improve appearance after loss of teeth for periodontal reasons

PMH: none relevant

o/e: both cast cobalt-chromium bases ill fitting; occlusal faults of dentures prevent intercuspal contacts on natural teeth (as shown in photographs of study casts)

Radiographs: full mouth radiographs taken by previous dentist

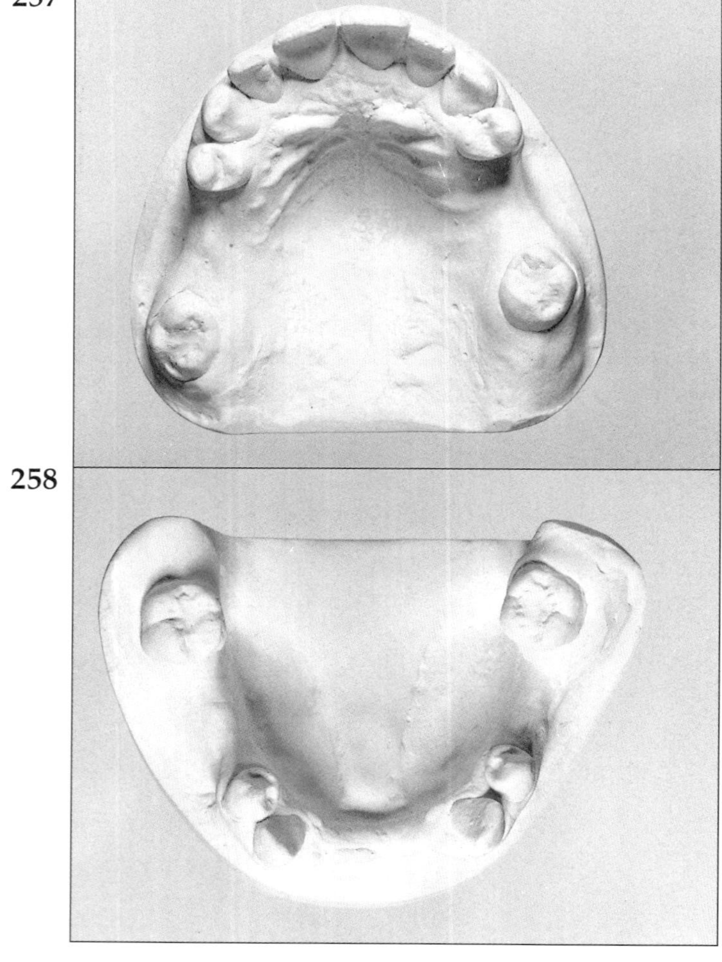

257

258

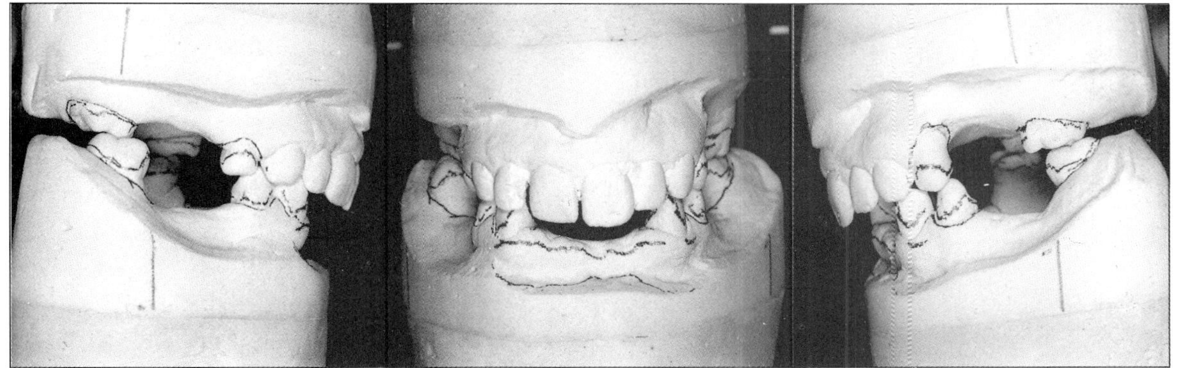

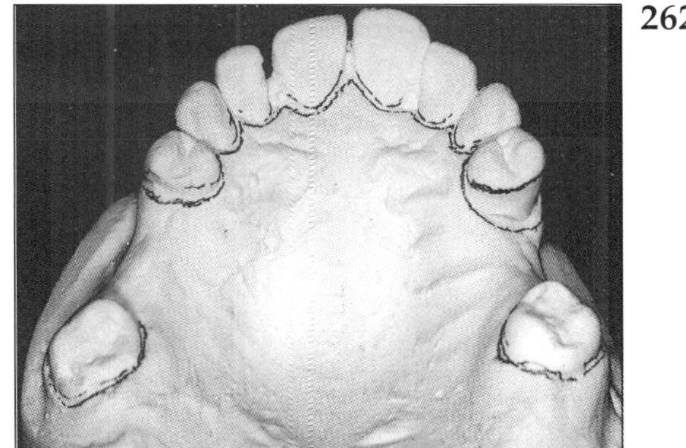

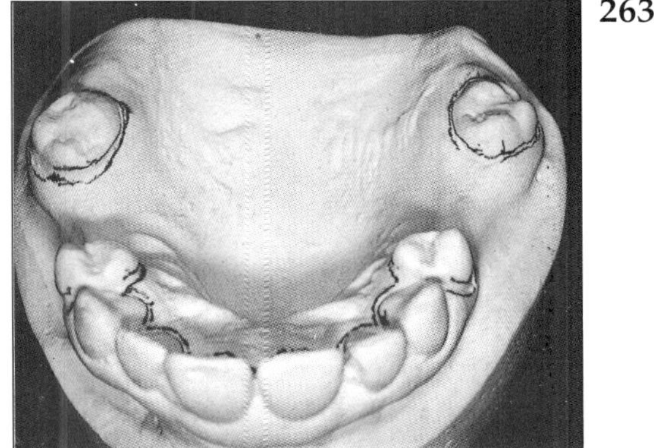

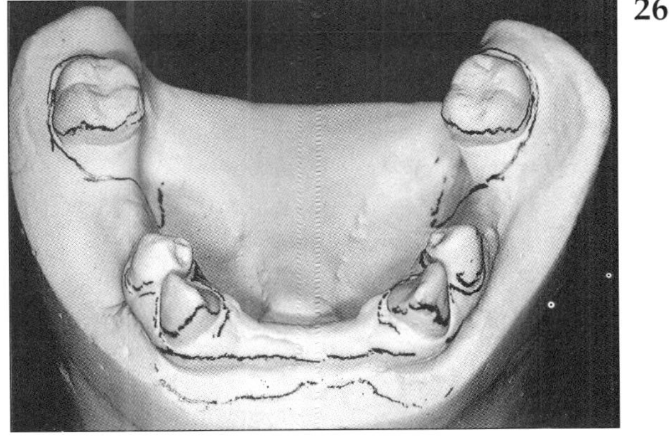

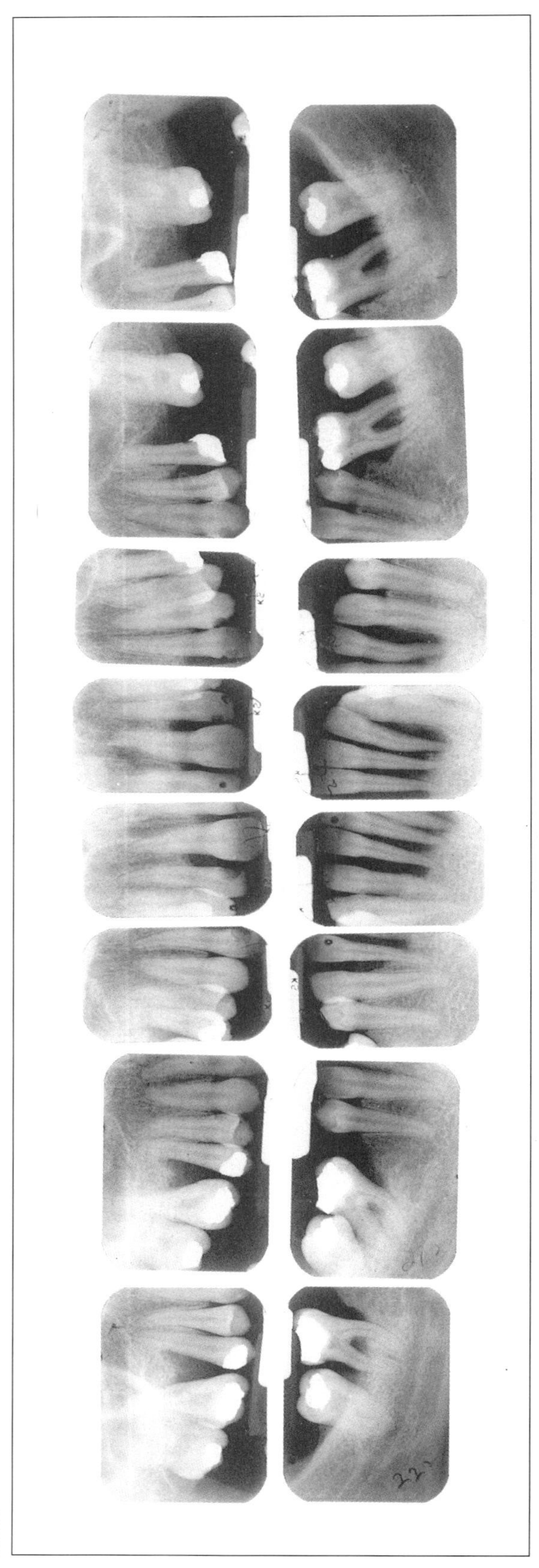

Treatment plan

Does this patient need RPD treatment?

The patient would like both upper and lower dentures to improve her appearance.

Dentally, the occlusion appears stable and a prosthesis is not necessary.

Treatment options

MAXILLA
- No denture.
- RPD (metal or acrylic).

MANDIBLE
- RPD (metal or acrylic)

Note: one generally accepted contraindication for fixed prosthodontics is poor oral hygiene and no patient can be allowed to ignore oral hygiene, which is basic to all dental treatment. It is arguable, however, that a well-made fixed prosthesis may have less plaque traps than a removable appliance, and could well be the treatment of choice in selected cases of poor oral hygiene (Watt and MacGregor, 1984). Nevertheless, for this patient, who has a poor periodontal prognosis, fixed prosthodontics is contraindicated.

Decision and treatment plan

This is influenced by the prognosis of the remaining dentition, finances and the patient's wishes.

- Stabilisation of periodontal condition.
- Restoration of carious lesions, incorporate an undercut in restorations on 27(DB) and 17(DB).
- Upper and lower RPD (cobalt-chromium).

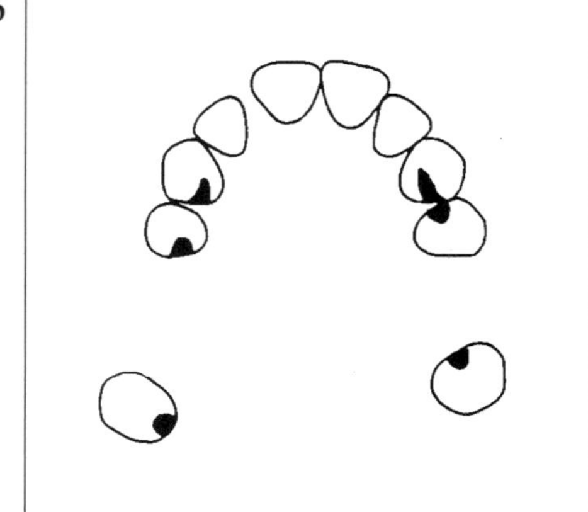

Fig 266 Support.

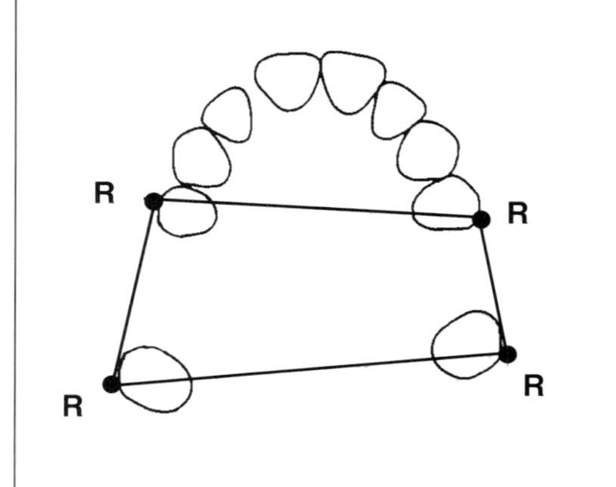

Fig 267 Retentive pattern.

Design

Maxilla

EDENTULOUS AREAS TO BE RESTORED
2 tooth supported.

SUPPORT
- Occlusal rests 17(P), 14(D), 24(M) and 27(M).
- Cingulum rests on 13 and 23 as supplementary support due to poor periodontal condition of 14 and 24.

RETENTIVE PATTERN
Rectangle between 14, 24, 27 and 17.

RETENTIVE UNITS
- 14 T-bar into very small B undercut (reciprocated by palatal plate).
- 24 I-bar into DB undercut (reciprocated by palatal plate).
- 17 short ring clasp into prepared DB undercut (reciprocated by palatal plate).
- 27 ring clasp into prepared DB undercut (reciprocated by occlusal rest).

CONNECTOR
Mid-palatal plate.

ACRYLIC ANCHORAGE
Mesh over edentulous areas.

TOOTH MODIFICATION
- Restorations of 17 and 27(DB) incorporating undercuts.
- Smooth areas for occlusal rests.

COMMENTS
Four retainers are needed because the undercuts are poor and guide planes would be of little help due to the very short clinical crowns of the molars.

Mandible

3 tooth supported.

Support
Occlusal rests 37(M), 47(M), 34(D) and 44(M) (to avoid distal occlusal contact).

Retentive pattern
Triangle between 37, 34 and 47 augmented by guide planes and occlusal rests on 44. The two retentive units on 37 and 47 will help to counteract the potential tissueward forces acting on the anterior base.

Retentive units
- 37 and 47 shortened ring clasps into DL undercuts make efficient use of survey line with minimum tooth modification (self-reciprocating).
- 34 I-bar into DB undercut (reciprocated by lingual plate).

Connector
Lingual plate.

Acrylic anchorage
Mesh over edentulous areas.

Tooth modification
- Smooth areas for occlusal rests.
- Guide planes on proximal surfaces of abutments.
- Lower survey line 37(MB) and 47(MB) to accommodate first (rigid) part of retainer.

Comments
Occlusal rests are not used on 37(D) and 47(D) due to occlusal contacts.

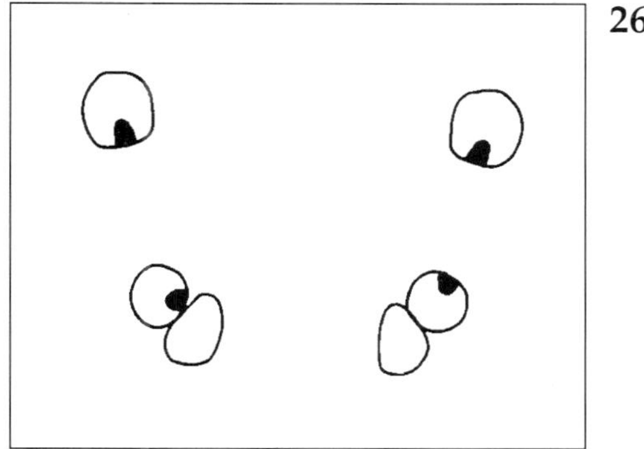

Fig **268** Support.

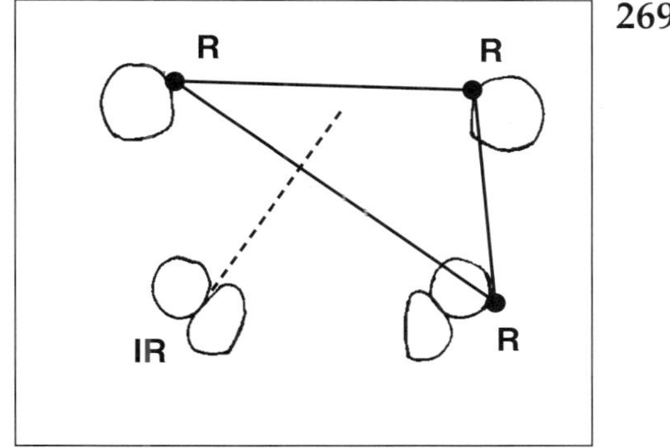

Fig **269** Retentive pattern.

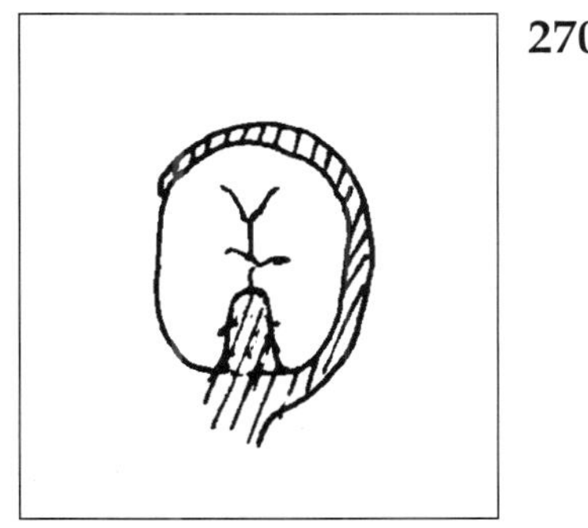

Fig **270** Shortened ring 37.

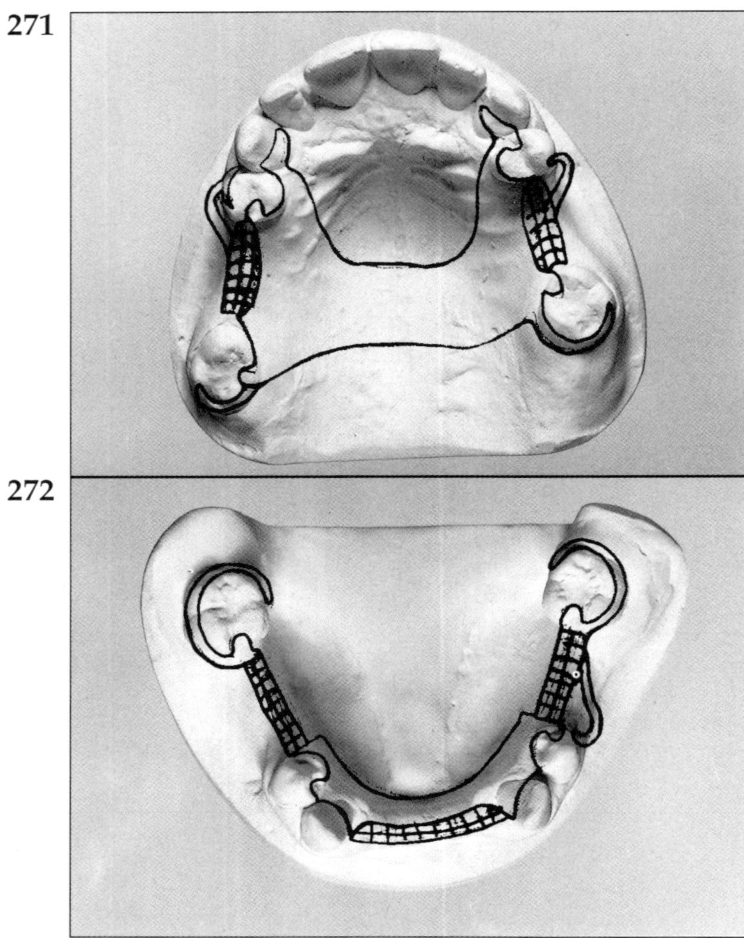

271

272

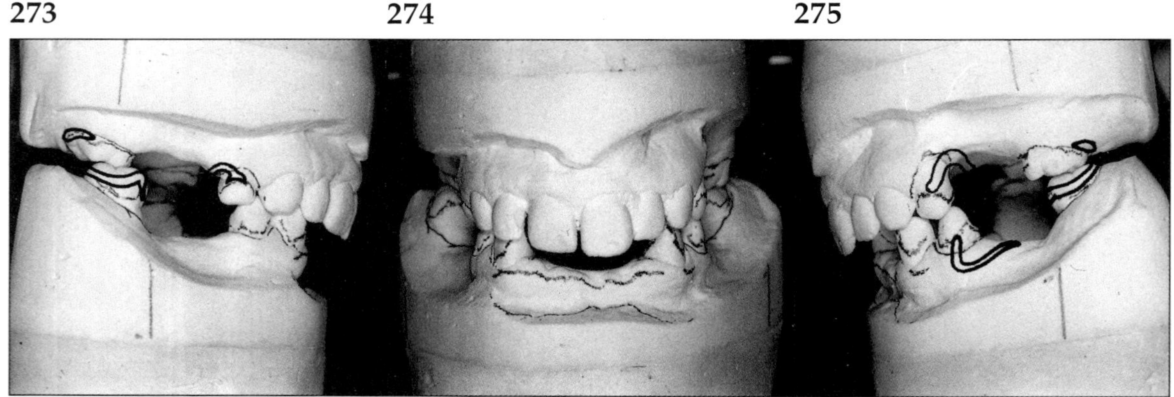

273   274   275

Patient No 10 (Figs 276–288)

History and examination

Name: C.C.R.
Sex: male

Age: 72 years
Occupation: retired stockbroker

c/o: worried about future of remaining teeth, especially upper; present partial dentures reasonably comfortable but lower partial denture not always worn

PDH: fairly regular attendance; present dentures about 7 years old

PMH: controlled hypertension

o/e: maxillary RPD – cobalt-chromium base; mandibular RPD – acrylic base; good oral health; remaining maxillary abutments good; periodontium and prognosis favourable

Radiographs: mandibular teeth only

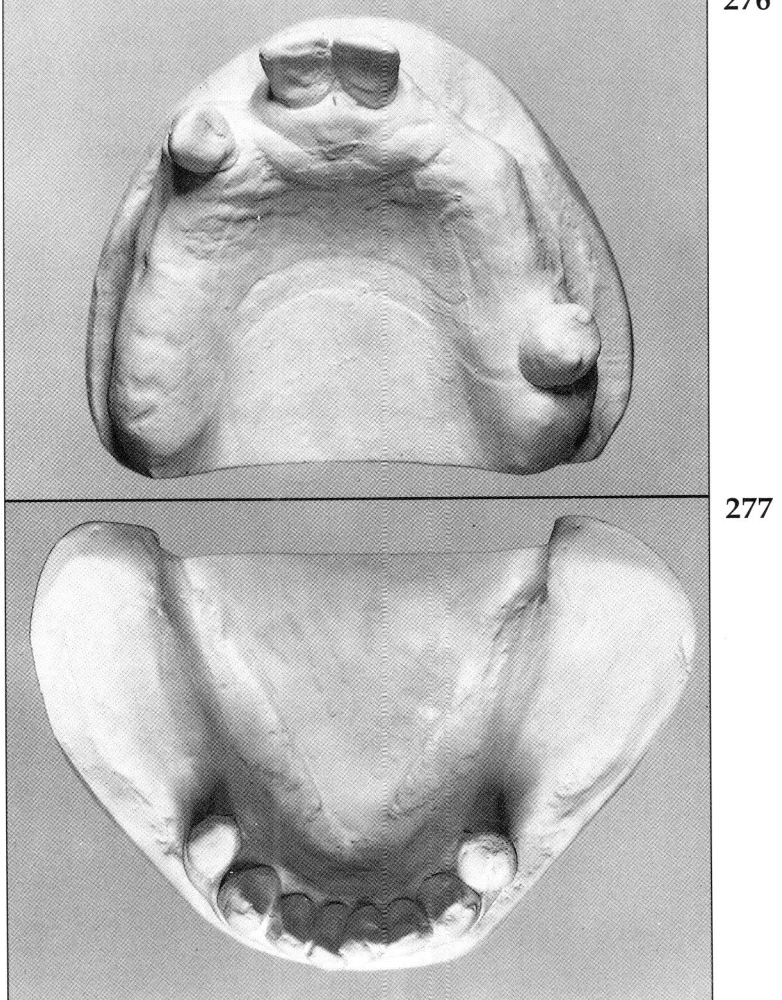

276

277

278 279 280

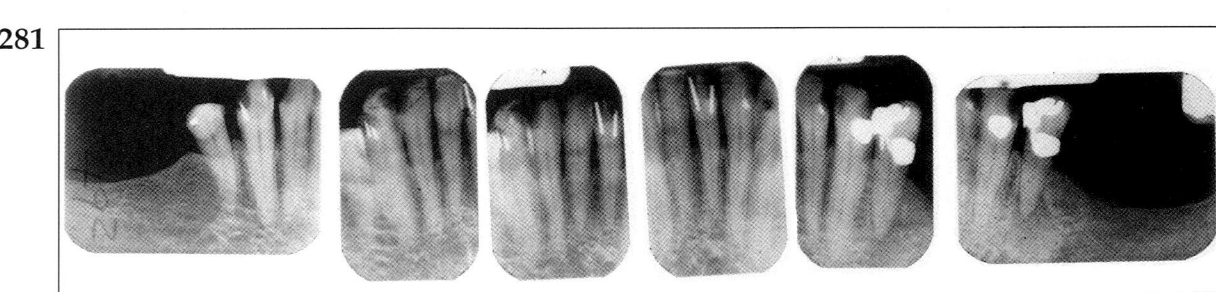

281

Treatment plan

Does this patient need RPD treatment?

The patient is concerned only about the upper jaw. He already has an upper denture but its appearance is poor.

Dentally, the arch is supported only to 34 and 44. Taking the patient's age into consideration, in the absence of symptoms, this may be adequate for his needs.

Treatment options

MAXILLA
- Adjust or reline the existing denture.
- New RPD with better aesthetics and preferably with palatal coverage to give more mucosal support (metal or acrylic).
- Root canal treatment 13, 11 and 21; reduce crowns and make an RP overdenture with or without attachments. By reducing the crown/root ratio and diverting the forces of the denture in a more axial direction, the roots of the teeth and, therefore, the alveolar bone would be maintained for a longer time.
- Root canal treatment 13, 11 and 21; reduce crowns; extract 28 and make a complete overdenture.
- Extract remaining teeth and make a complete denture.

Note: with fewer than six teeth remaining, RPD treatment is compromised. Both retention and support pose problems. If the decision is made to extract the remaining maxillary teeth it is essential that a satisfactory mandibular RPD is made and worn so that the occlusion is balanced. Without this the complete denture may well be a failure.

MANDIBLE
- Nothing.
- Adjust existing denture to be more comfortable.
- New metal RPD having thinner (and therefore more comfortable) lingual plate.

(Absence of radiographs is an obvious drawback in the definitive treatment plan of this case and this omission must be rectified before treatment commences.)

Decision and treatment plan

This is influenced by finance, periodontal health and the patient's wishes.

- Preparation and restoration of abutment teeth.
- Upper and lower cobalt-chromium RPDs.

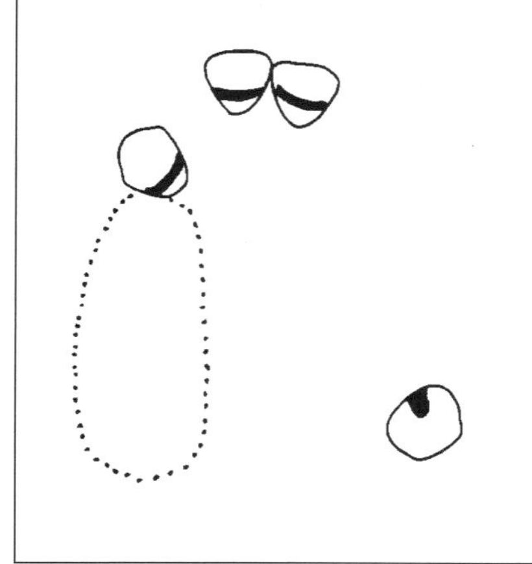

Fig **282** Support.

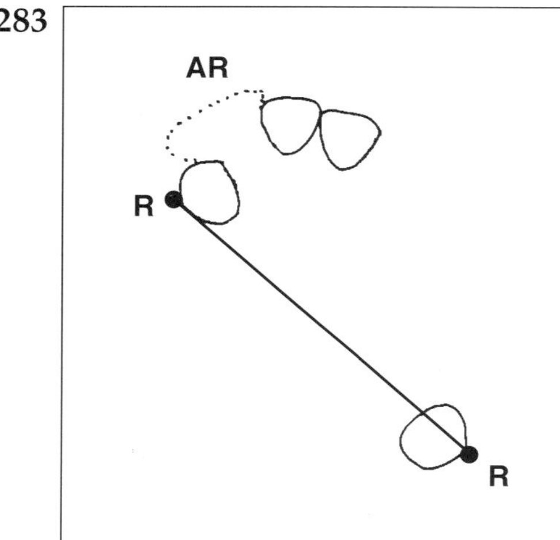

Fig **283** Retentive pattern.

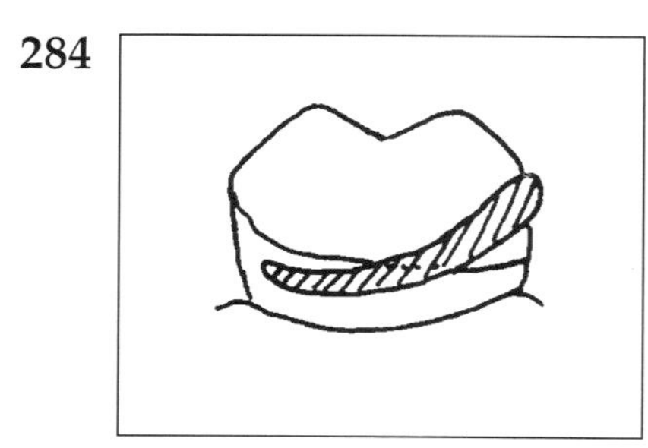

Fig **284** 'Ideal' undercuts provided by the crown.

Design

Maxilla

Edentulous areas to be restored
- 2 tooth supported.
- 1 tooth and mucosa supported.

Support
- Full veneer crowns with prepared cingulum rest seats, 13, 11 and 21.
- Full crown with prepared occlusal rest seat 28(M).
- Maximum coverage of DEB area.

Retentive pattern
Straight line between 13 and 28, augmented by wide labial flange 12 and 22, and by guide planes on all abutments.

Retentive units
- 28 circumferential into DB undercut (reciprocated by plate).
- 13 I-bar into DB undercut (reciprocated by plate).

Connector
Ring connector with collets around denture teeth.

Acrylic anchorage
- Pin 12.
- Loops in other edentulous areas.

Tooth modification
Full veneer crowns prepared with path of insertion planned. Guide planes, rest seats and undercuts for retainers are all integral parts of the crowns.

Comments
Two diagonal retainers are barely sufficient for this design. The result relies on the precision of the guiding surfaces and the extra retention offered by the labial acrylic flanges.

Full palatal coverage would have given more mucosal support, but was omitted due to the patient's wishes.

Mandible

EDENTULOUS AREAS TO BE RESTORED
2 tooth and mucosa supported.

SUPPORT
- Occlusal rests 34(ML) and 44(ML).
- Maximum extension of edentulous areas, with altered cast technique.

RETENTIVE PATTERN
Straight line between 34 and 44.

RETENTION
I-bars 34(B) and 44(B) (reciprocated by minor connectors of rests).

CONNECTOR
Lingual bar.

ACRYLIC ANCHORAGE
Mesh over edentulous areas with tissue stops.

TOOTH MODIFICATION
Full veneer crowns 34 and 44.

COMMENTS
Crown fabrication is essential as the anatomy of the natural abutments (34 and 44) is unsuitable for the rest, plate and I-bar of this design (RPI system, page 43).

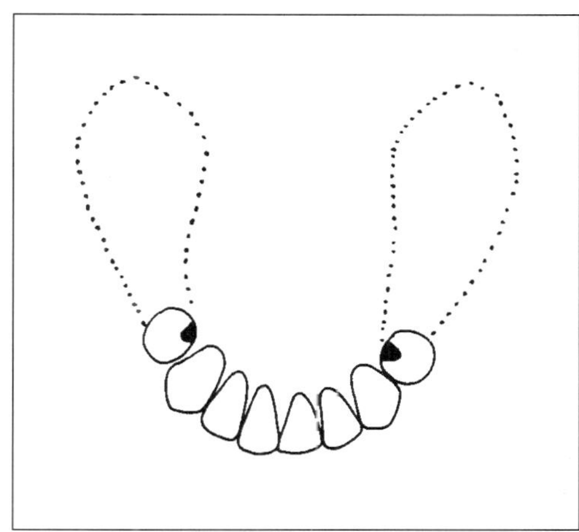

285

Fig **285** Support.

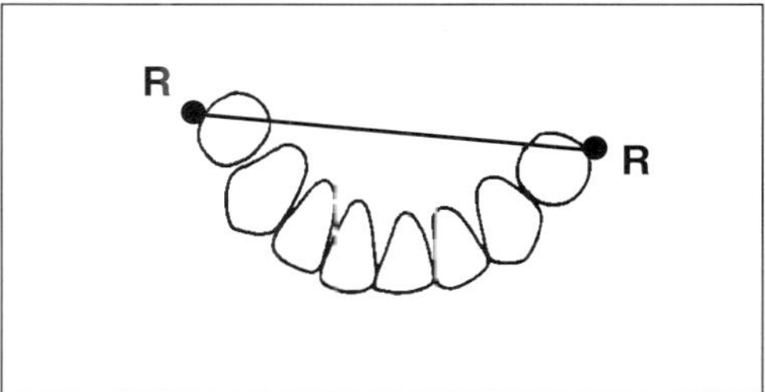

286

Fig **286** Retentive pattern.

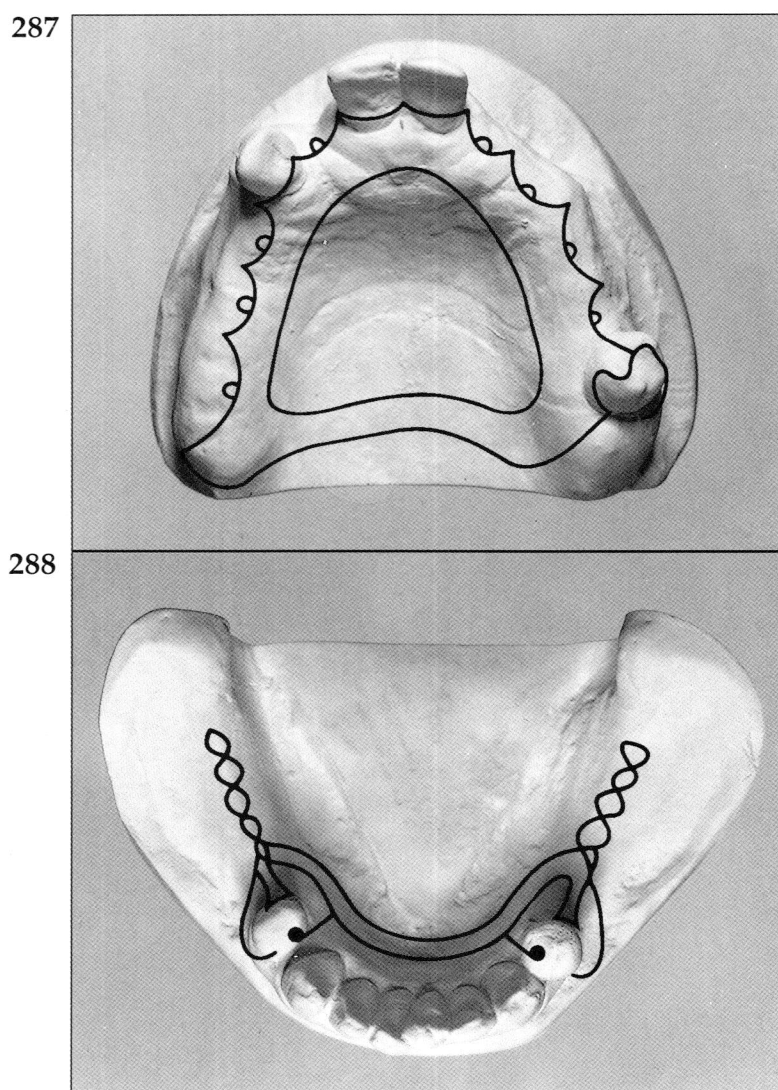

Patient No 11 (Figs 289–301)

History and examination

Name: I.T.W. *Sex:* male

Age: 44 years *Occupation:* solicitor

c/o: present RPD, made about 3 years ago, has poor appearance

PDH: maxillary anterior teeth lost some years ago, possibly due to apical infection; regular attendance

PMH: none relevant

o/e: maxillary acrylic RPD with gum-fitted incisors, shade incorrect; good oral hygiene; slight gingival damage palatal maxillary first molars

Radiographs: nil

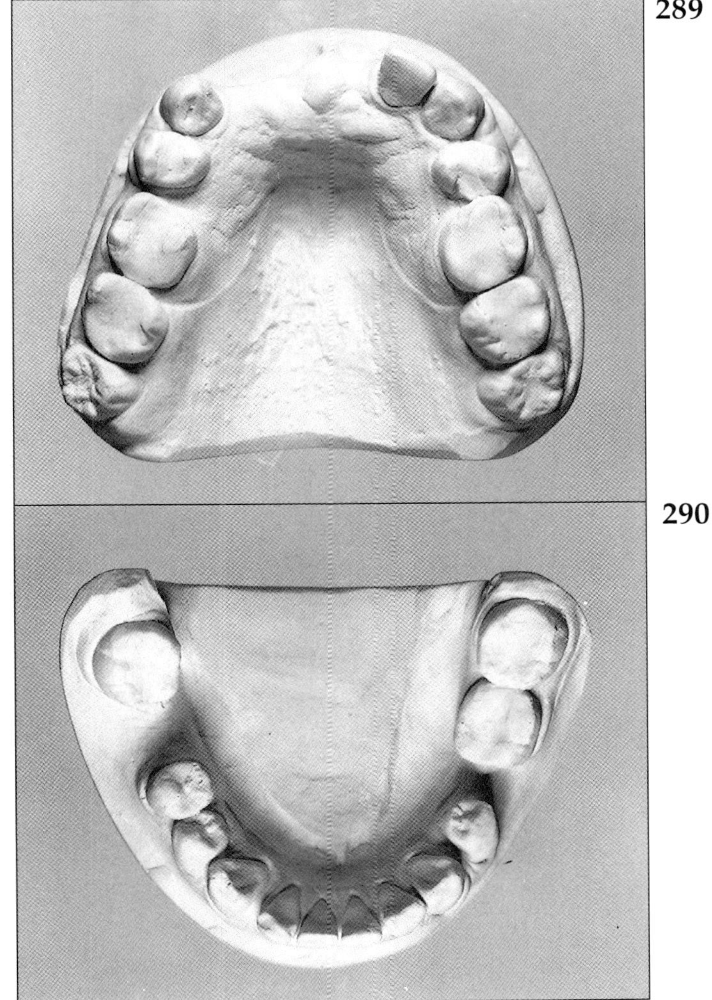

289

290

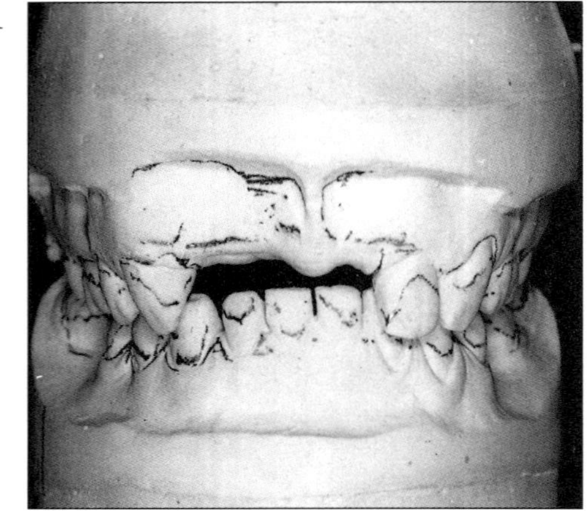

291

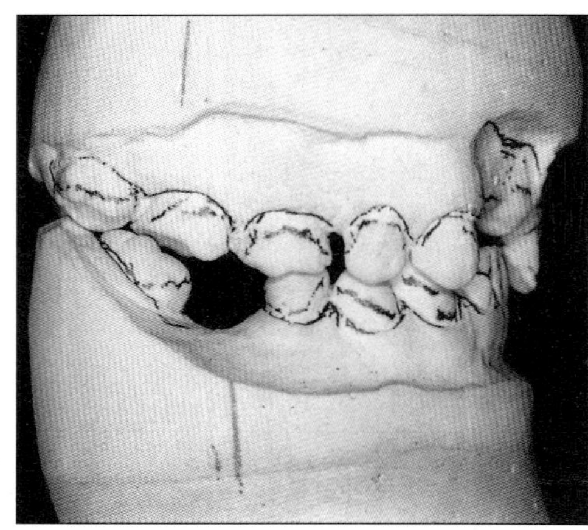

292

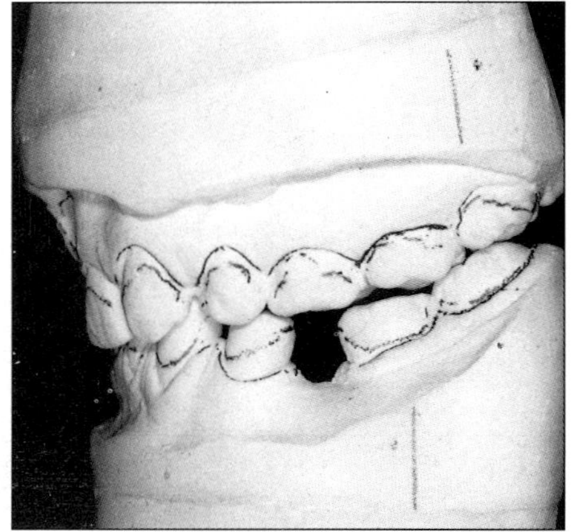

293

Treatment plan

Does this patient need RPD treatment?

The patient needs a maxillary prosthesis for aesthetics.

Dentally, the arch is stable.

Treatment options

MAXILLA
- Osseointegrated implants supporting fixed restoration.
- RPD (metal or acrylic) with flange to restore lost contour.

MANDIBLE
- Nothing.
- Fixed prostheses restoring 35 and/or 46.
- RPD (metal or acrylic).

Note: absence of radiographs is an obvious drawback in the definitive treatment of this case and this omission should be rectified if at all possible.

Decision and treatment plan

This is influenced by finances, the patient's wishes and gingival/mucosal irritation caused by the present denture.

- Extract 18 which is overerupted and is a potential source of occlusal interference.
- Upper RPD (cobalt-chromium).
- No mandibular prosthesis.

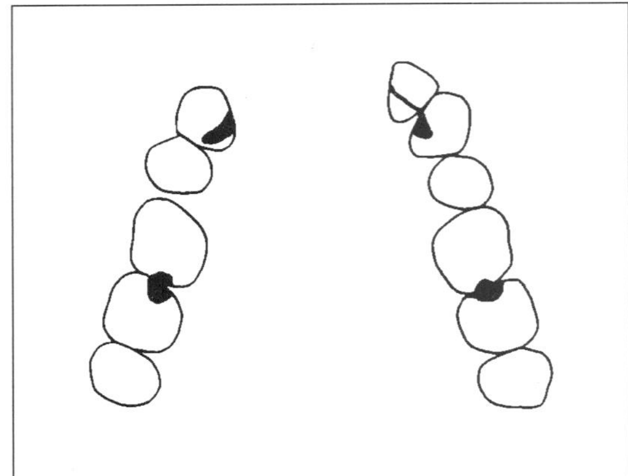

Fig **294** Support.

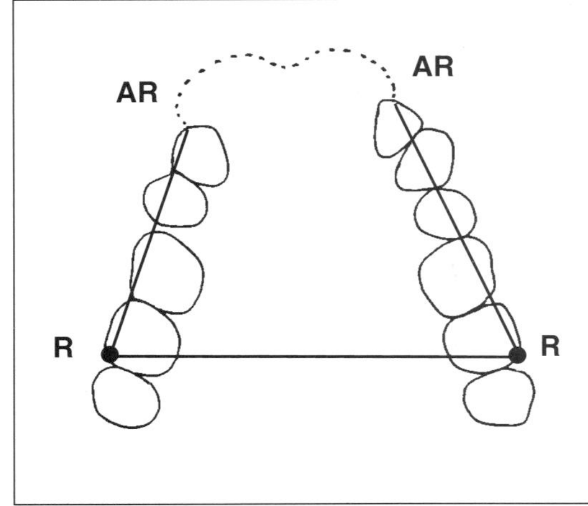

Fig **295** Retentive pattern.

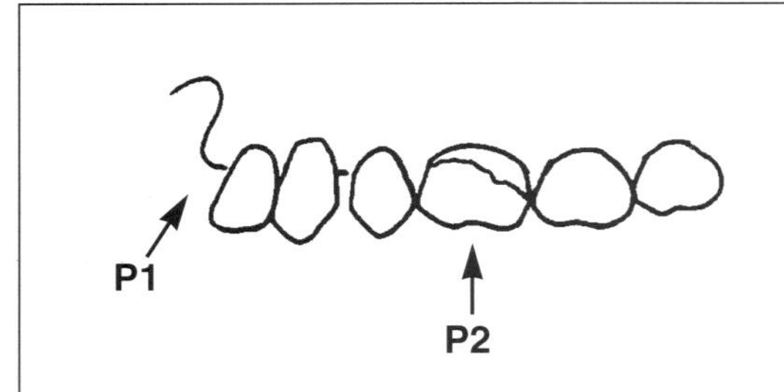

Fig **296** Rotational path of insertion.

Design

Maxilla

EDENTULOUS AREAS TO BE RESTORED
1 tooth supported.

SUPPORT
- Occlusal rests 17(M) and 27(M) with tiny extensions on to distal surface of 16 and 26 to create marginal ridges.
- Cingulum rest 13 and 23(M).

Note: 22 is spoon shaped and not suitable for a rest seat.

RETENTIVE PATTERN
Tetragon between 17, 13, 22 and 27. Rotational path of insertion.

RETENTIVE UNITS
- Retainers.
- 17 and 27 circumferential into DB undercuts (reciprocated by palatal arms entering disto-palatal fissures to make them less perceptible to the tongue).
- Rigid sections of denture in mesial undercuts of 13, 22.

CONNECTOR
Anterior palatal plate with collets round 12, 11 and 21, the position of which must be determined before laying down a wax pattern for the cast framework. Palatal extensions to retainers on the molars.

ACRYLIC ANCHORAGE
Loops or mesh.

TOOTH MODIFICATION
Occlusal rests will stand proud on flat, uncontoured amalgam restorations if the rest seats are not prepared, but such preparations may weaken the amalgams. A degree of compromise is necessary. The edges of the rests should merge as far as possible with the edges of the prepared seats.

The retainers must enter the undercuts with respect to both the path of insertion, that is, the cast tilted, and the path of displacement , that is, the occlusal plane horizontal, in order to be retentive.

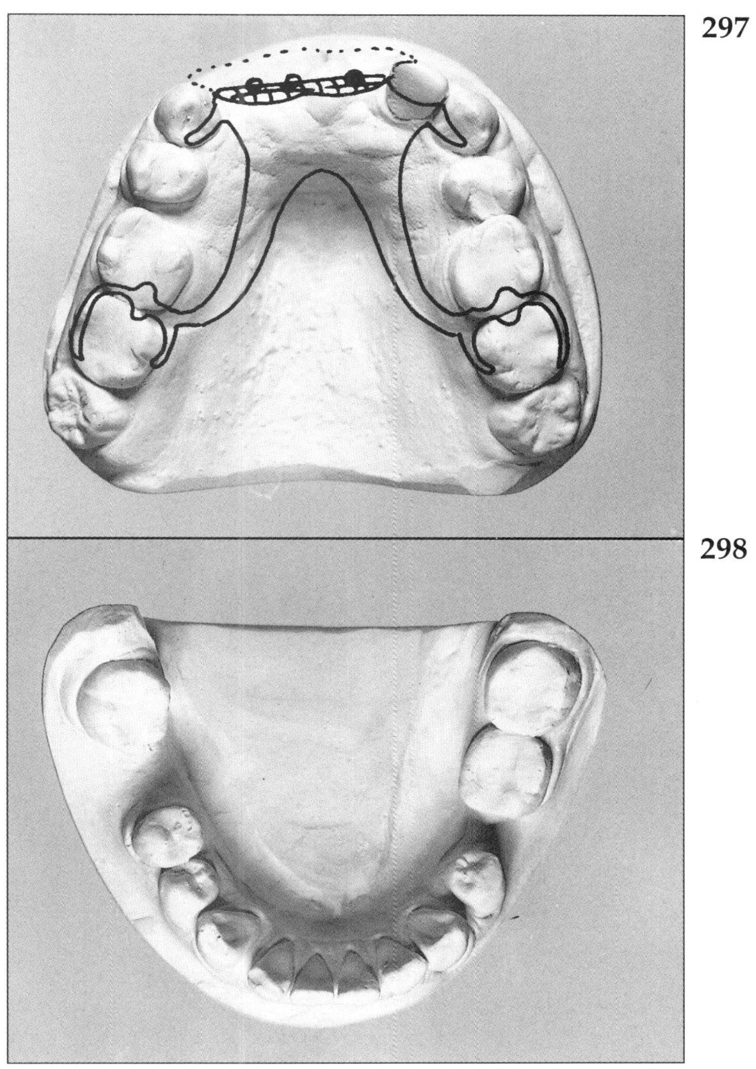

297

298

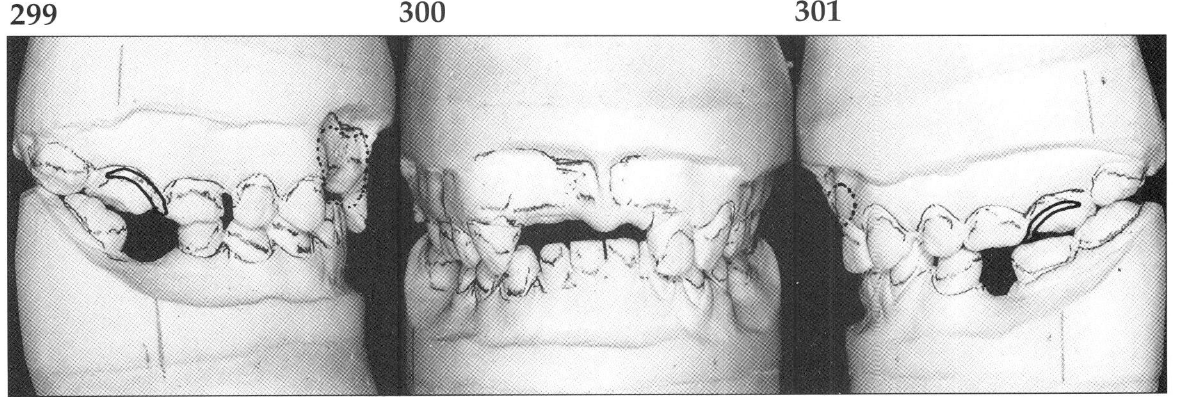

299 300 301

Patient No 12 (Figs 302–317)

History and examination

Name: E.N.F.　　*Sex:* male

Age: 50 years　　*Occupation:* fruit salesman

c/o: told by family to 'get something done about your teeth'; slightly concerned about wearing away of front teeth

PDH: infrequent dental treatment; partial lower denture made some years ago but uncomfortable and never worn

PMH: alcohol intake slightly above average

o/e: typical tooth surface loss (TSL); restorations of good quality; oral hygiene good; gingival state excellent

Casts are shown in: closed intercuspal position (Figs **304–306**); approximate acceptable occlusal face height (OVD) (Figs **307–309**)

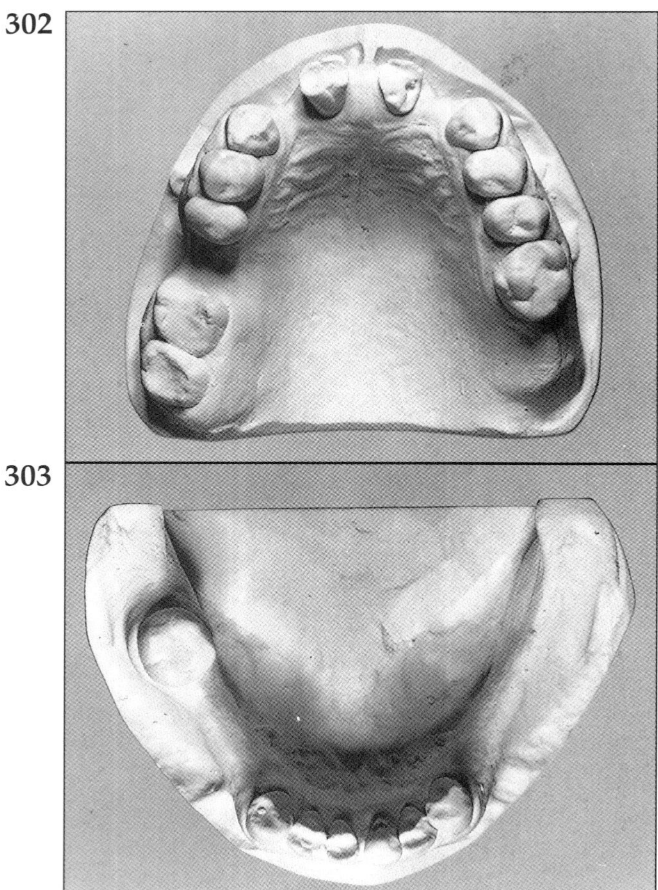

302

303

304 305 306

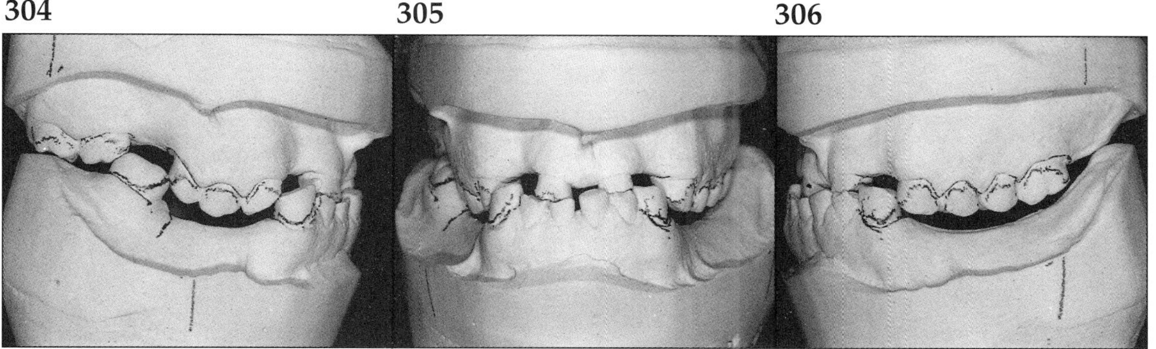

307 308 309

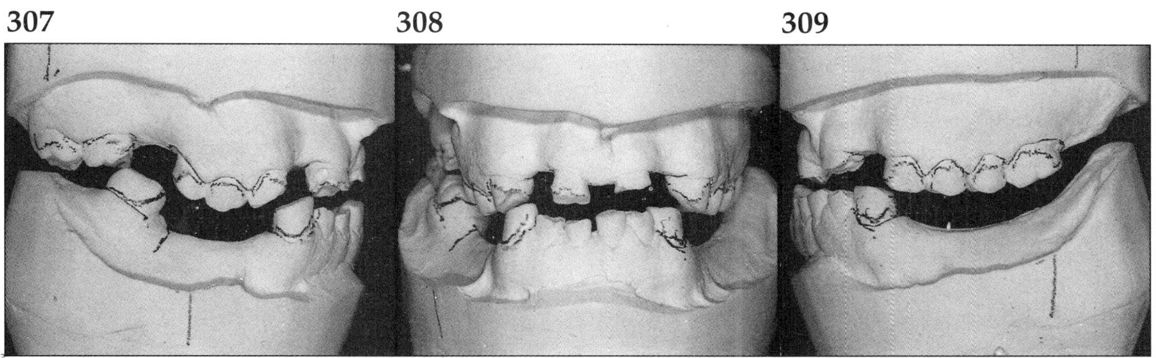

Treatment plan

Does this patient need RPD treatment?

The patient is not very dentally aware but is willing to please his family's concern about his upper anterior teeth.

Dentally, the arch has collapsed. Posterior support is needed. 18 and 15 have overerupted carrying the alveolus with them. The collapse is causing wear on the anteriors.

Treatment options

MAXILLA
- Fixed prosthesis restoring edentulous areas and OVD.
- Crowns on 11, 13 and 21 and RPD restoring edentulous areas. This is a poor option. The patient would probably not wear the RPD once the upper anteriors were aesthetically restored.
- RP overdenture (metal).

MANDIBLE
RPD (metal) with or without restoration of lower anteriors.

Decision and treatment plan

This is influenced by radiographs, finances and the patient's possible lack of compliance in wearing the lower RPD due to lack of perceived benefit and left DEB.

- Smooth sharp enamel edges on 11 and 21 and construct an acrylic splint to an acceptable OVD with tooth-coloured acrylic over 11 and 21 (page 135).
- Monitor the patient's compliance, oral hygiene, etc, before proceeding further. Note that this is the most difficult time for the patient. Therefore the splint must be as small and as comfortable as possible.
- Root canal treatment on 11 and 21 and reduce to gingival level. Restore the canal opening with glass-ionomer cement (GIC). Adjust the splint accordingly by adding tooth-coloured acrylic or denture teeth.
- Restore the incisal edges of 32, 31, 41 and 42. Reduce the height of 43 (mesial tip), that is, restore the lower incisal plane. Adjust the splint accordingly.
- Reduce the DB cusps of 47. Adjust the splint.
- Restore the buccal surfaces of 33 and 43 with indentations for retainers.
- Maxillary RP overdenture (cobalt-chromium). Mandibular RPD (cobalt-chromium).
- Instruct the patient in the use of NaF 2 per cent on 11 and 21 daily.

Design

Maxilla: splint

Acrylic covers the occlusal and incisal surfaces to restore occlusal integrity.

The splint is retained by circumferential clasps on 18, 13, 23 and 26. The position of the clasps ensures that retention will not be compromised when the splint is adjusted.

Maxilla: denture

2 tooth supported.

- Occlusal rests on all posterior teeth to maintain the occlusal plane even if the lower RPD is not worn.
- Grid over 17(M), 15(DP) and 13(M).

Triangle between 18, 13 and 26.

- 18 and 26 circumferential clasps into DB undercut (reciprocated by palatal arm).
- 13 circumferential clasp into MB undercut (reciprocated by palatal plate).

'Horseshoe' plate.

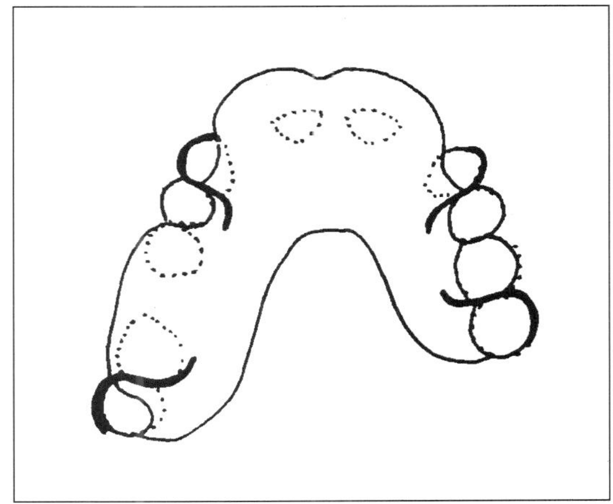

Fig **310** Splint.

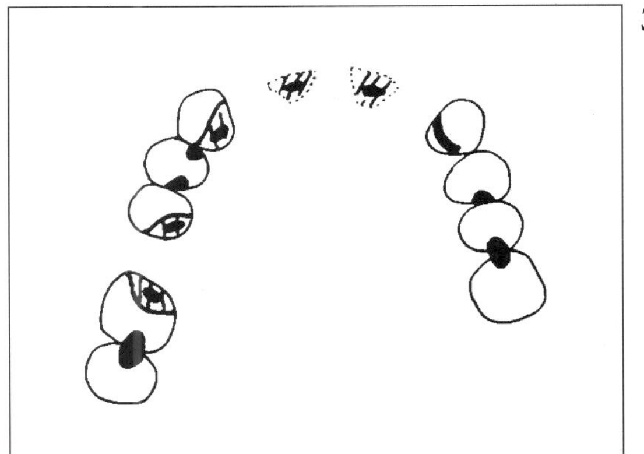

Fig **311** Support.

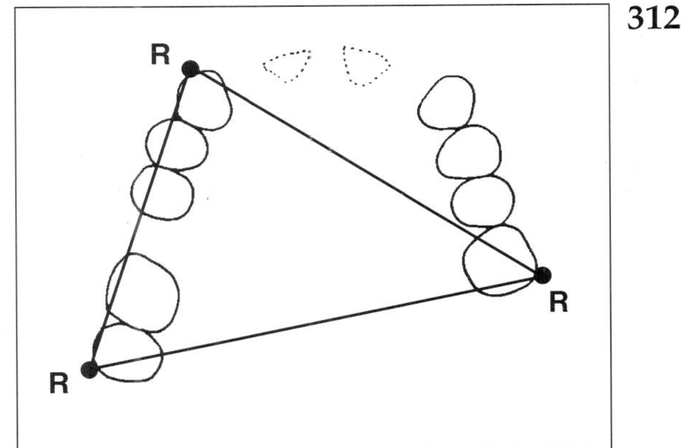

Fig **312** Retentive pattern.

313

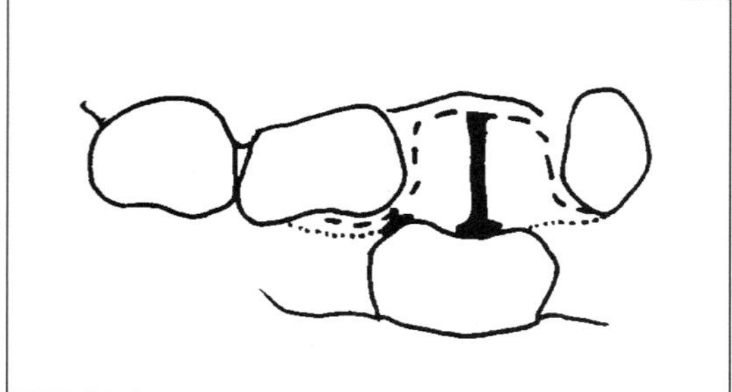

Fig **313** Studs maintain occlusal contact.

Acrylic anchorage
Extends over occlusal surfaces of 17(M), 15(D) and 13(M) with small studs giving occlusal contact (page 34)

Tooth modification
- Smooth areas for occlusal rests.
- Guide planes 17(M) and 15(D).

Comments
The mesh on the mesiopalatal surface of 13 has to be carefully designed to avoid aesthetic problems.

Mandible

Edentulous areas to be restored
1 tooth supported.
1 tooth and mucosa supported.

Support
- Occlusal rest 47(M).
- Cingulum rests 33 and 43.
- Maximum mucosal coverage of DEB.

Retentive pattern
Triangle between 47, 43 and 33.

Retentive units
- 47 ring clasp into DL undercut (self-reciprocating).
- 33 and 43 I-bars into prepared buccal undercuts (reciprocated by lingual plate).

Connector
Lingual plate.

Acrylic anchorage
Mesh over edentulous areas with tissue stop on DE area.

Tooth modification
Lower survey line 47(MB) to allow first (rigid) part of ring clasp to engage.

Comments
It is very likely that this patient will not wear his lower RPD. It is therefore important to ensure that his perceived benefit (pleasing his family by improved aesthetics) and the dental benefit of restoring occlusal integrity are linked together in the upper RPD.

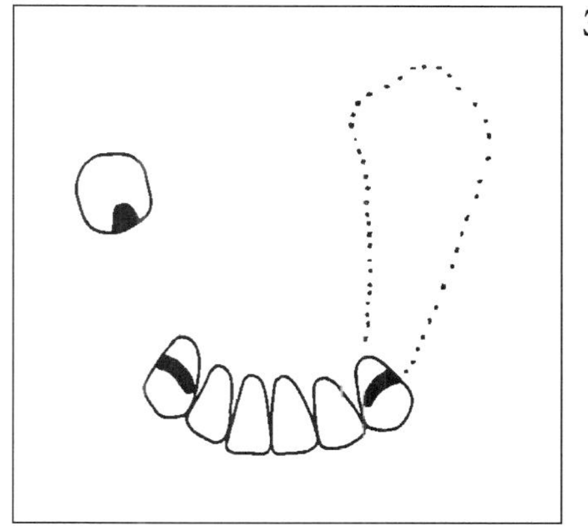

314

Fig 314 Support.

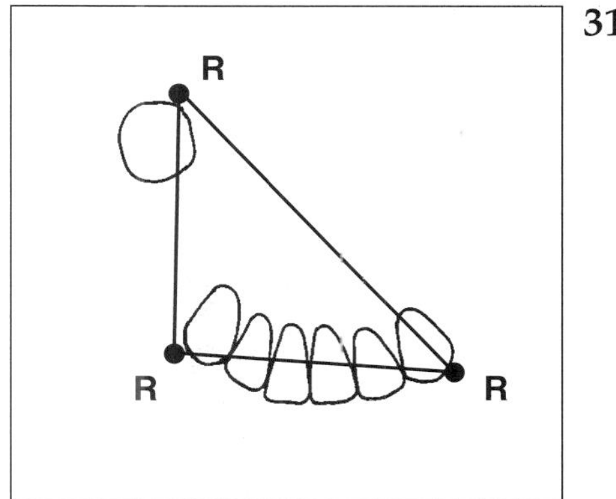

315

Fig 315 Retentive pattern.

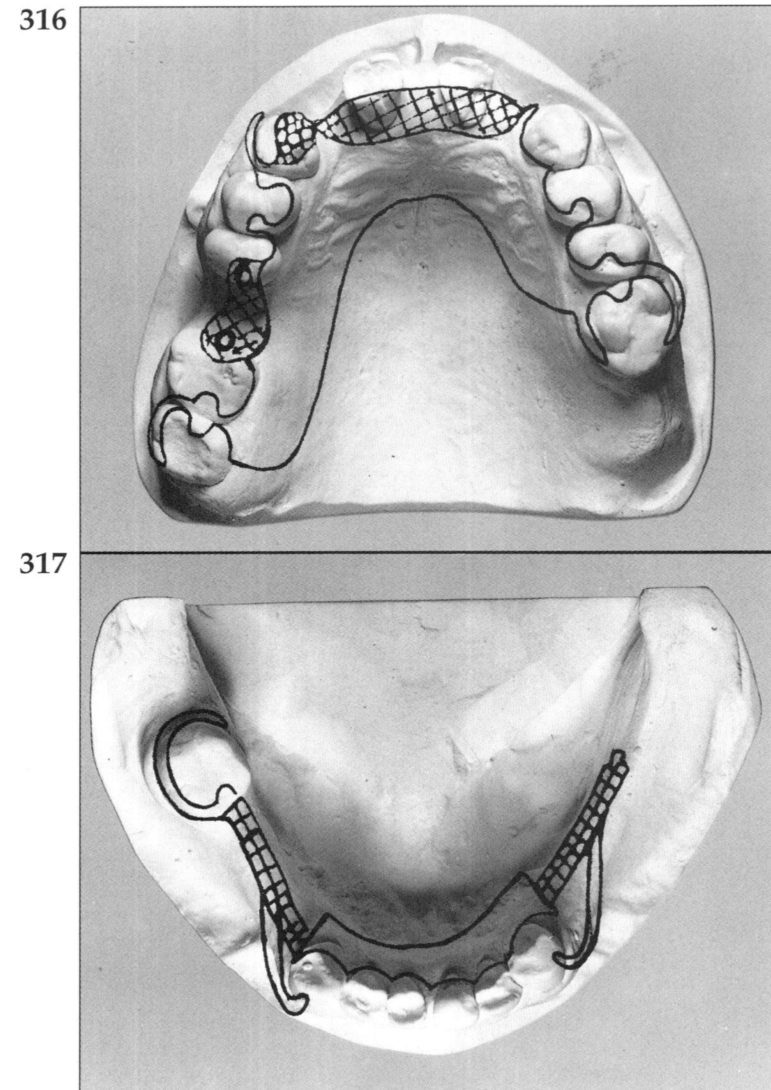

Patient No 13 (Figs 318–338)

History and examination

Name: T.C. *Sex:* male

Age: 47 years *Occupation:* bricklayer

c/o: wearing down of teeth

PDH: fairly frequent dental attendance; lengthening of upper anteriors attempted with pinned restorations; no denture experience

PMH: none relevant

o/e: marked TSL; previous restorative treatment of posterior teeth; oral hygiene good; vitality of maxillary anteriors negative

Radiographs: full mouth intra-oral (note bone density)

Casts shown in: closed 'tooth contact' position; open at acceptable occlusal face height

318   319   320

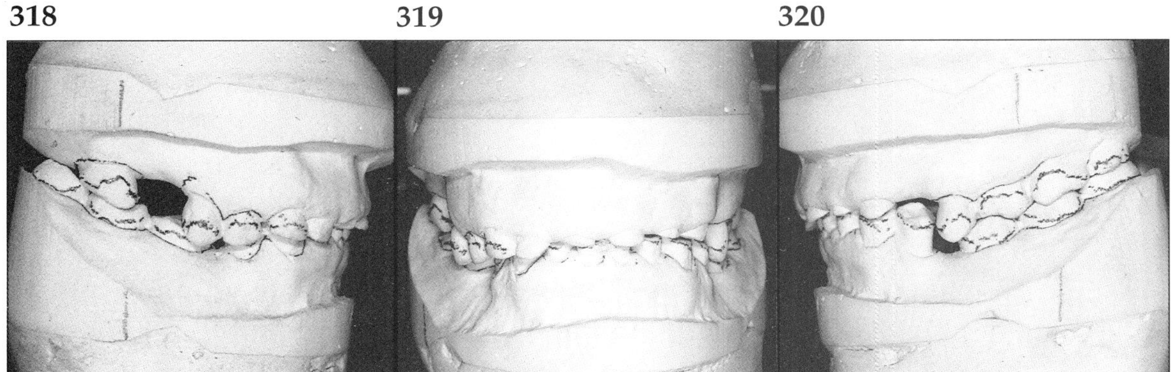

321   322   323

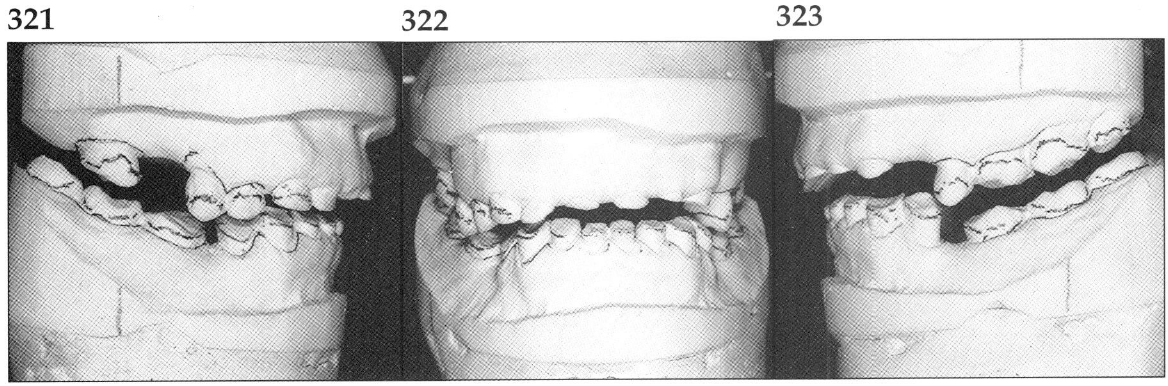

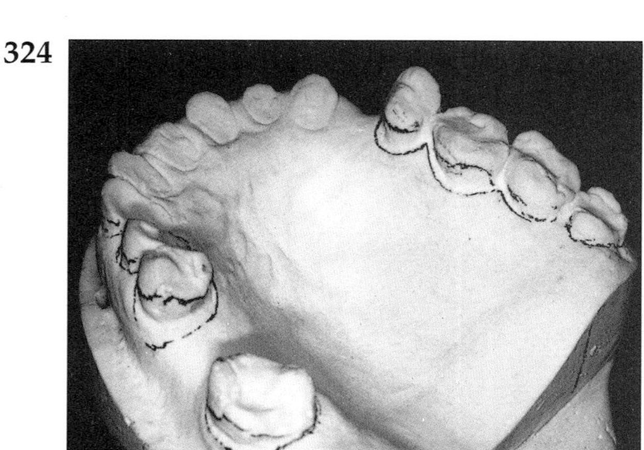

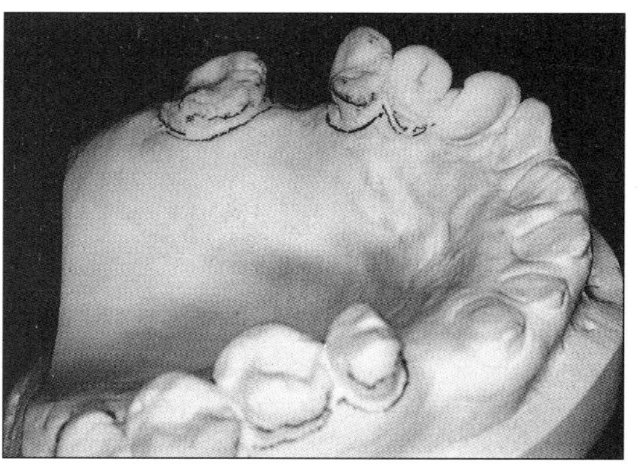

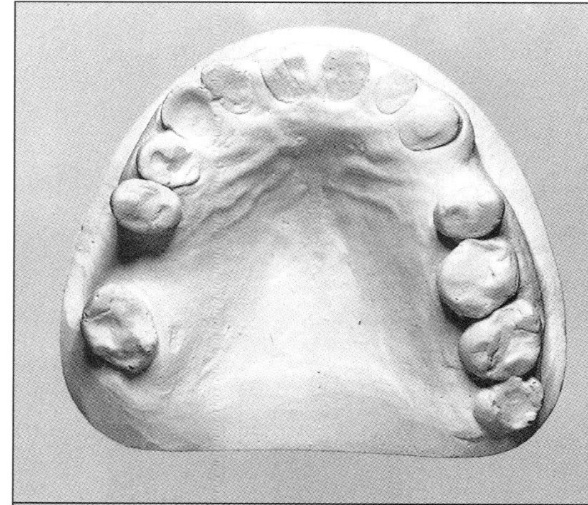

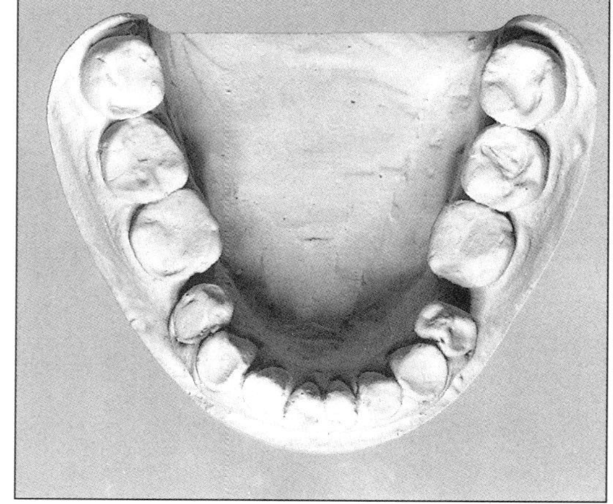

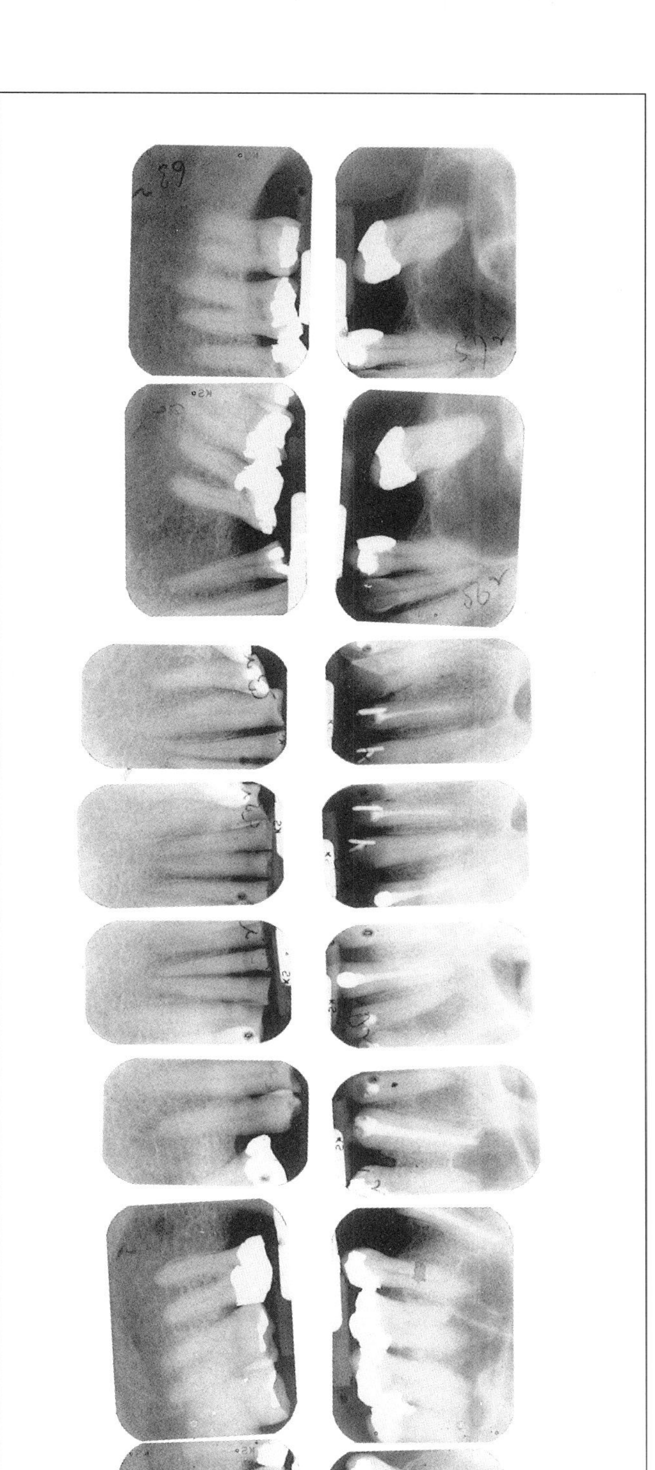

Treatment plan

Does this patient need RPD treatment?

The patient is concerned about wearing down his teeth.

Dentally, the occlusion has collapsed due to tooth wear, probably of thegotic origin.

Treatment options

- Restore OVD with fixed restorations.
- Restore OVD with a combination of restorations and RPD bearing in mind that the occlusion must be stable with no, one, or both dentures *in situ* (see page 13).

Decision and treatment plan

This is influenced by finances:

- Smooth sharp edges of the maxillary and mandibular anteriors and commence endodontic treatment of 13 (11 and 22 could also be treated endodontically, but are to be extracted because finances are limited). 12, 21 and 23 are already root filled.
- Construct a maxillary splint to correct OVD using tooth-coloured acrylic over maxillary anteriors (Fig **334**). Monitor the patient's reactions and adjust accordingly.
- Extract 48. Complete endodontic treatment of 13 closing off canal(s) with GIC.
- Restore posterior teeth with amalgam. Gold would be more desirable but finances are limited:
  - restore the mandibular molars to a desirable level (Fig **335**); adjust the splint accordingly;
  - restore the maxillary molars to provide posterior contact; cut the splint away from the posterior teeth, that is, convert it into a temporary RPD.
  - restore mandibular anteriors with composite; adjust the splint.
- Restore the maxilla with an RP overdenture.
- Construct a new splint to be worn at night and replace as necessary.

Design

Maxilla: splint

Michigan design (Fig **334**).

Maxilla: denture

Edentulous areas to be restored
2 tooth supported.

Support
- Occlusal rests 17(M), 15(D), 26(D) and 27(M).
- Root faces 13, 12 and 23.

Retentive pattern
Triangle between 17 and 27 and attachment on root face 21.

Retentive units
- 17 and 27 ring clasps into DB undercut (self-reciprocating).
- 21 intraradicular attachment.

Connector
'Horseshoe'.

Acrylic anchorage
- Pins for 16, 13, 12, 11, 22 and 23.
- Mesh over saddle areas carried to middle of root faces and cut away around 21 for attachment part.

Tooth modification
- Occlusal rest seats (incorporated in the restorations).
- Guide planes 17(M), 15(D), 14(M) and 25(M).

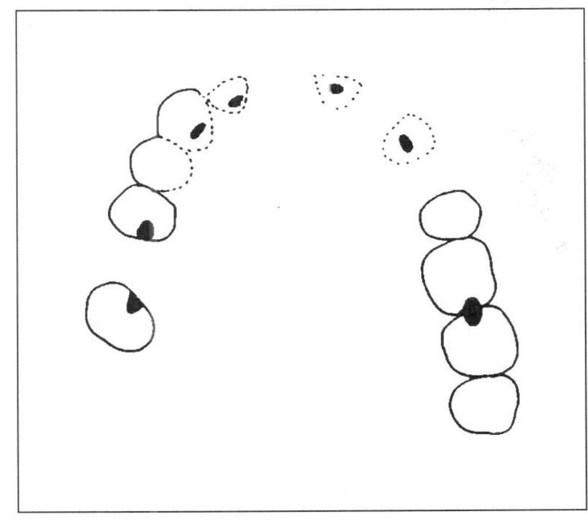

Fig **330** Support.

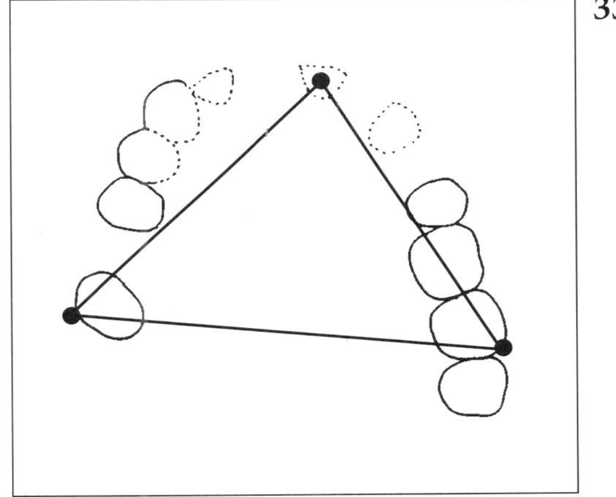

Fig **331** Retentive pattern.

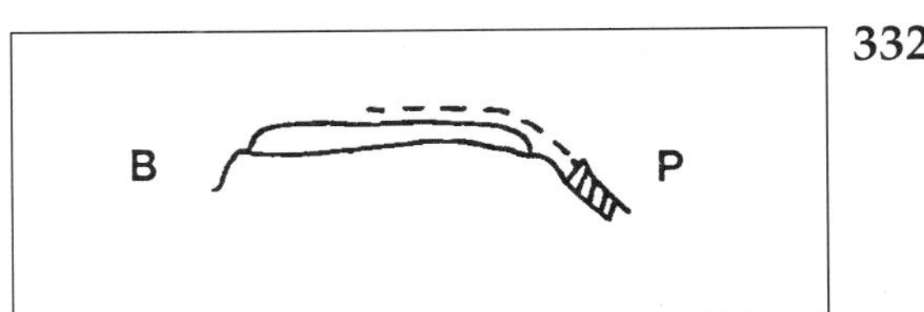

Fig **332** Mesh is carried to the middle of the root face of 13, 12, 23.

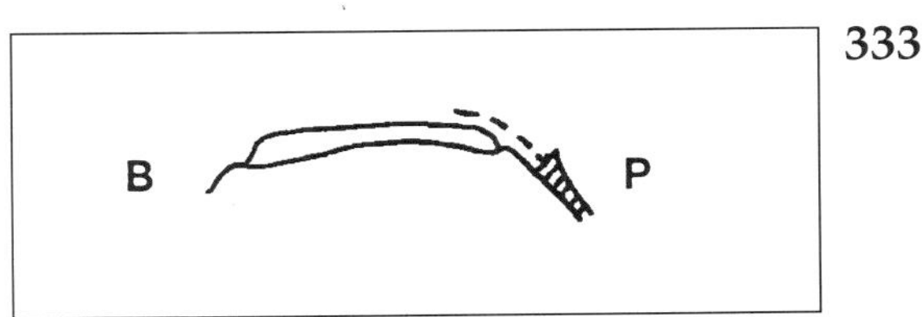

Fig **333** Mesh is cut away from the root face of 21.

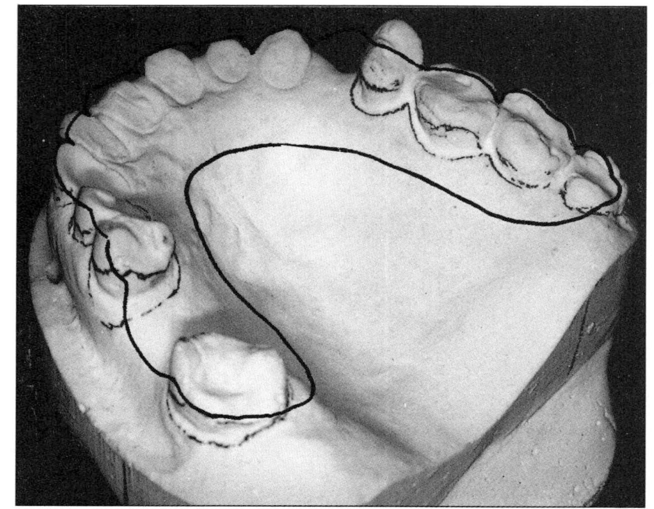

334

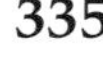335

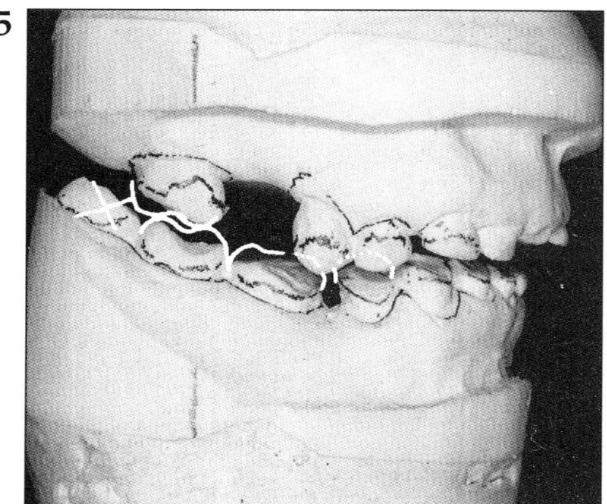

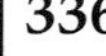336

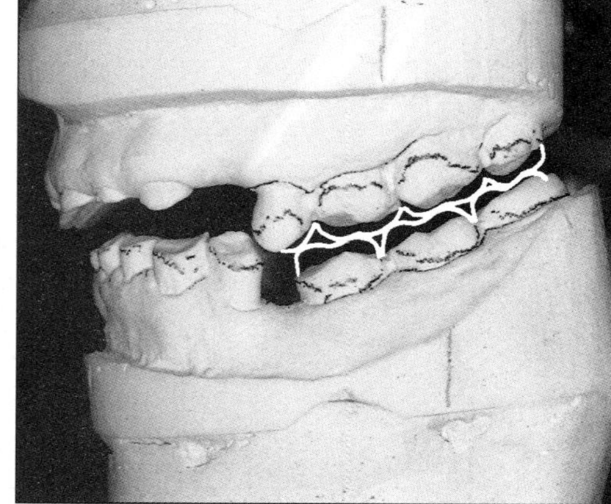

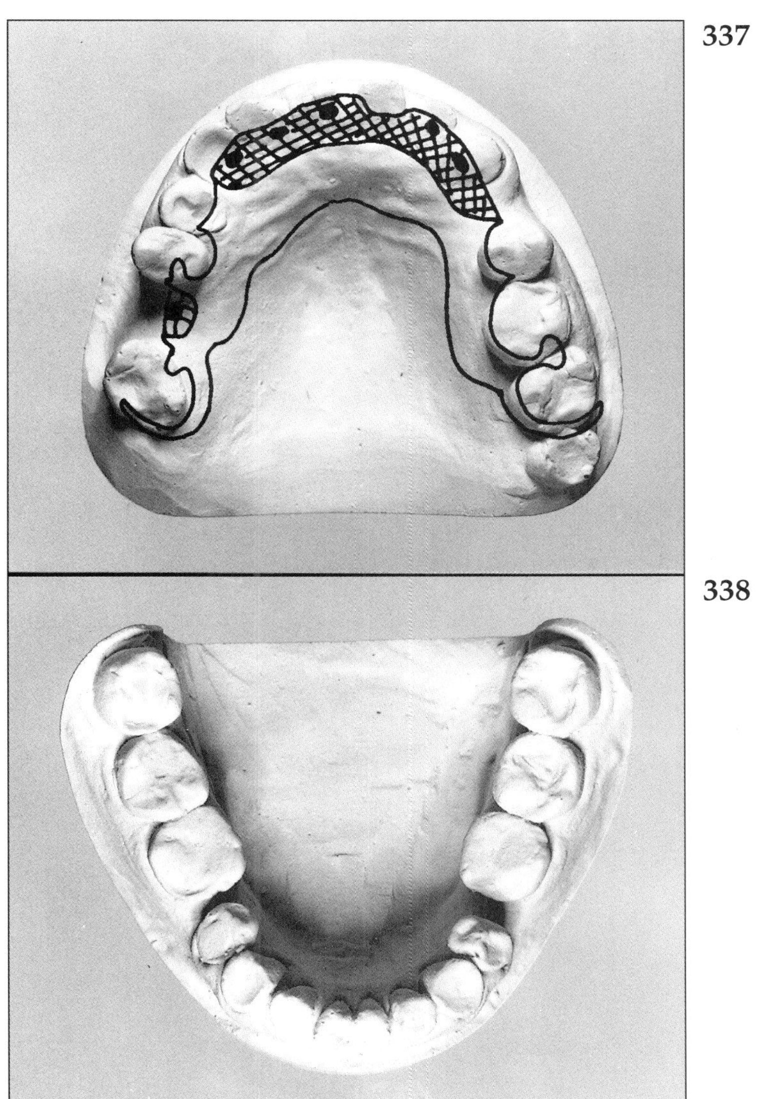

Patient No 14 (Figs 339–352)

History and examination

Name: H.J.J.   *Sex:* female

Age: 63 years   *Occupation:* housewife

c/o: present acrylic dentures 4 years old and frequent breakages; teeth wearing away

PDH: teeth extracted from time to time; never remembered any fillings; various dentures over the years but usually broke fairly soon

PMH: mild rheumatoid arthritis

o/e: marked TSL, no obvious aetiology; occlusion totally collapsed

Radiographs: orthopantomograph

Casts shown: in closed position; at approximate correct OVD

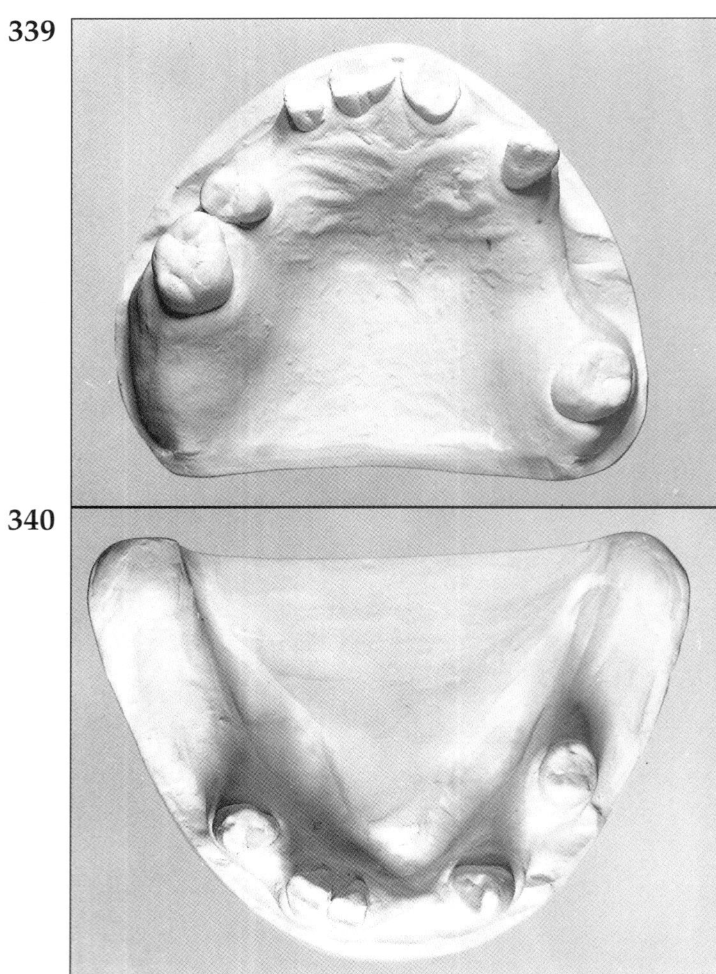

339

340

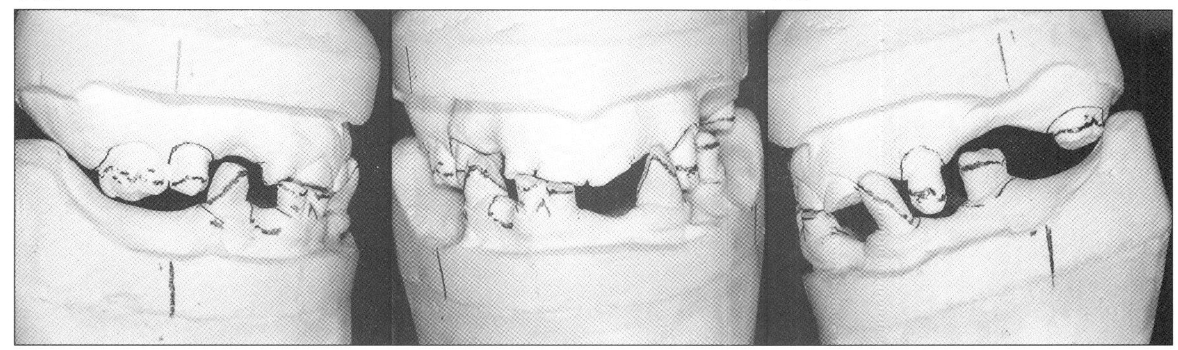

341
342
343

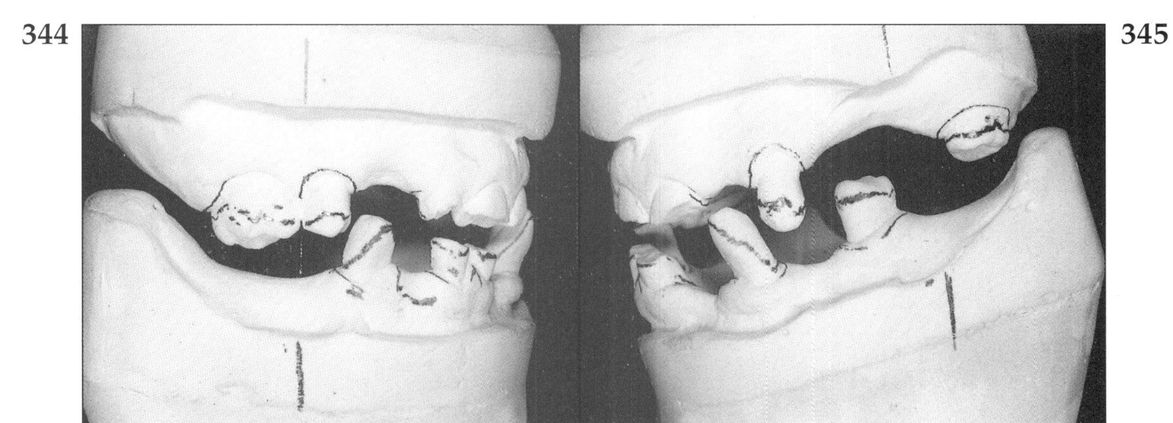

344
345

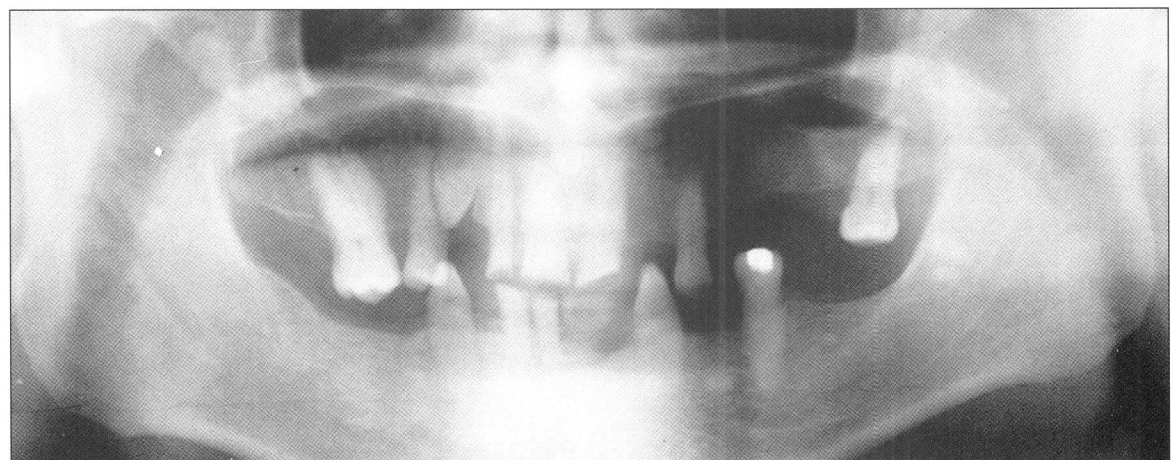

346

Treatment plan

Does this patient need RPD treatment?

The patient wants to restore her appearance.

Dentally, the occlusion has collapsed and overerupted teeth are causing occlusal interference.

Treatment options

MAXILLA
* A combination of fixed and removable prosthesis.
* Restorations of anteriors with crowns or composites and RPD (metal).

MANDIBLE
* A combination of fixed and removable prosthesis with possible crowns/composites on lower anteriors.
* RPD (metal or acrylic).
* Complete overdenture over canine root faces.

Decision and treatment plan

This is influenced by finances and the patient's lack of commitment to complex dental treatment.

* Investigate retained roots and unerupted 13. No pathology. Tell the patient and leave *in situ*.
* Reduce the length of 23 and 16 (palatal cusp). Construct a splint over maxillary teeth using tooth-coloured acrylic over anterior teeth, and denture teeth in anterior edentulous areas at correct OVD.
* Extract 41, 42 and 35 and replace with an immediate (acrylic) RPD, adjusting both the upper splint and lower denture to give a desirable occlusal plane. Pay particular attention to correct peripheral extensions and to buccolingual tooth placement (as for complete dentures). The denture has plastic teeth to minimise wear against opposing dentition/restorations (*see* Fig **352**).
* Root canal treatment of 33 and 43.
* Restore 12, 11 and 21 with composite, cut away splint as necessary.
* Reduce 33 and 43 to the gingival margin and convert an RPD into a complete overdenture (with or without intraradicular attachments).
* Construct an upper RPD (cobalt-chromium) (design 2) and reline lower overdenture.

Designs

Maxilla

EDENTULOUS AREAS TO BE RESTORED
3 tooth supported.

SUPPORT
- Occlusal rests 16(M), 15(M) and 27(M).
- Cingulum rests 12, 21 and 23.

RETENTIVE PATTERN
Triangle between 16, 12 and 27 augmented by cingulum rests and guide planes on proximal surfaces.

RETENTIVE UNITS
- 16 and 27, ring clasps into DB undercuts (self-reciprocating).
- 12 wrought gold I-bar into DB undercut (reciprocated by palatal plate).

CONNECTOR
Mid-palatal plate.

ACRYLIC ANCHORAGE
Posts in anterior edentulous areas as required (see below).

TOOTH MODIFICATION
- Smooth areas for occlusal rests and cingulum rests.
- Guide planes on proximal surfaces as determined for anterior edentulous areas (see below).

COMMENTS
- The retentive pattern would have been better between 16, 23 and 27 (bigger triangle). However, 23 is periodontally compromised and probably healthier without a retainer.
- The anterior edentulous areas are too large for 1 tooth replacement and too small for 2 teeth. Clinical trials will show whether diastemas or lapping of teeth is desirable and will influence the position of posts and preparation of guide planes approximating these edentulous areas.

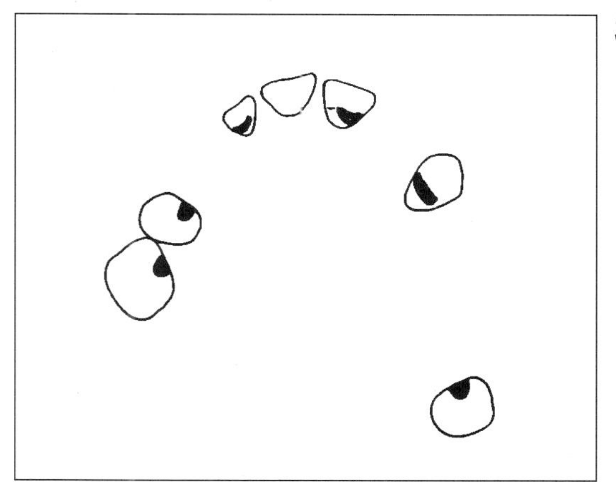

Fig **347** Support.

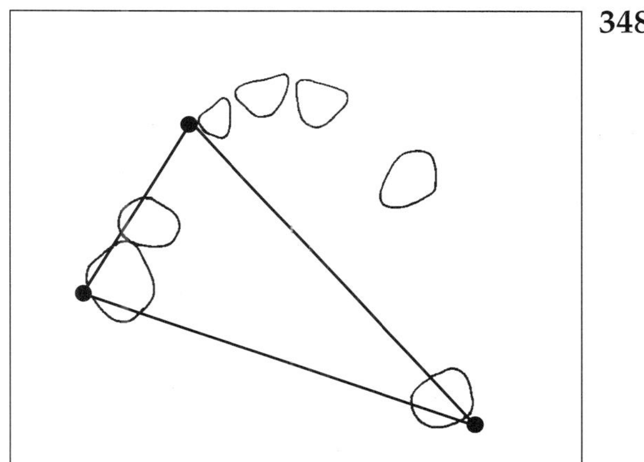

Fig **348** Retentive pattern.

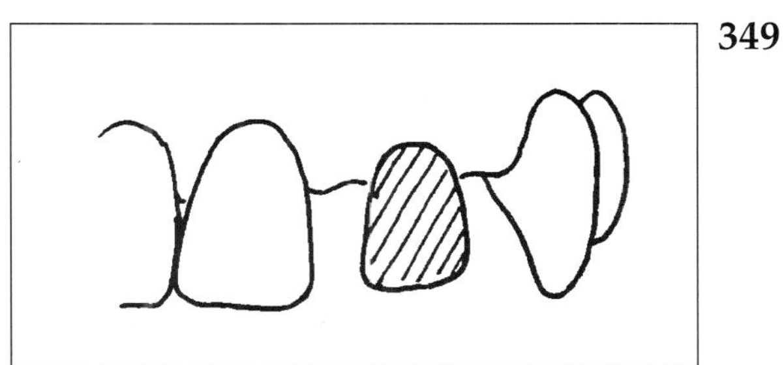

Fig **349** Anterior edentulous area. One tooth replacement.

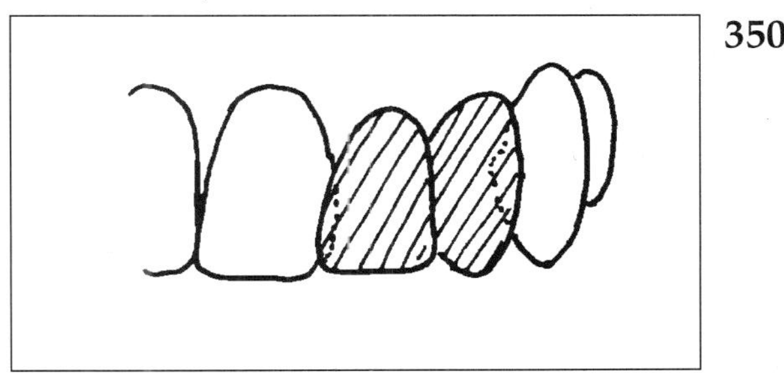

Fig **350** Anterior edentulous area. Two tooth replacement.

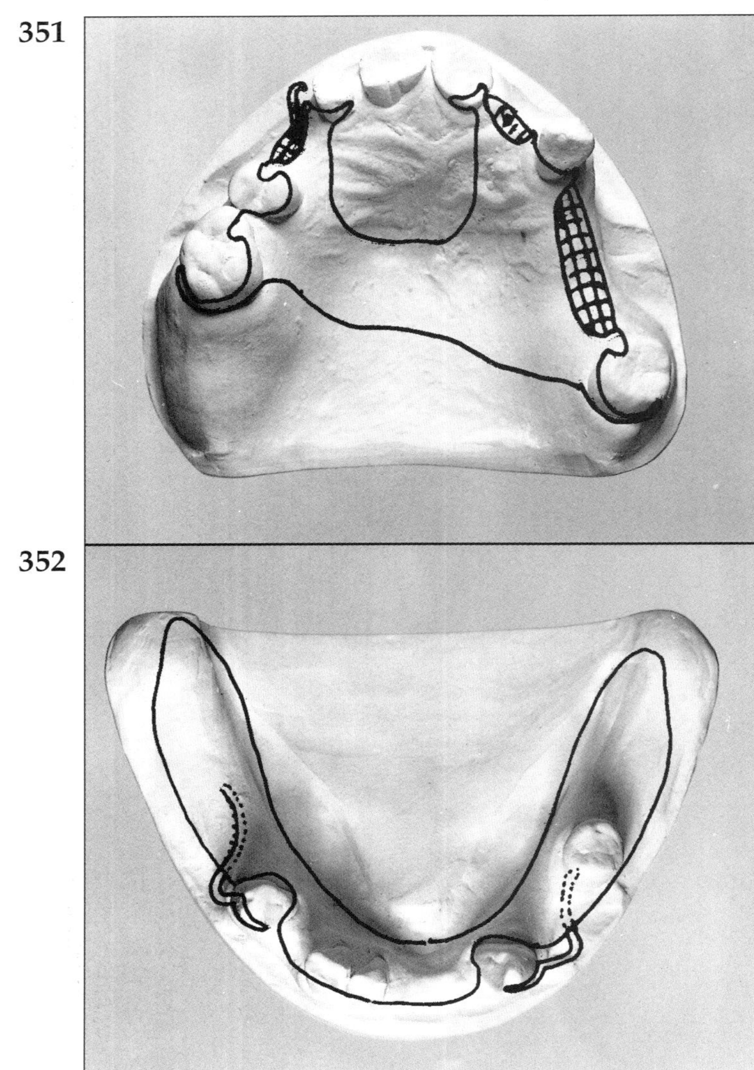

Design Errors (Figs 353–361)

The following show hypothetical designs for patients 2 and 12. Assume that no tooth modification has been done. Each design has at least five errors, any one of which could jeopardise the success of treatment. These errors are listed on pages 152 and 154.

Patient no 2

353   354

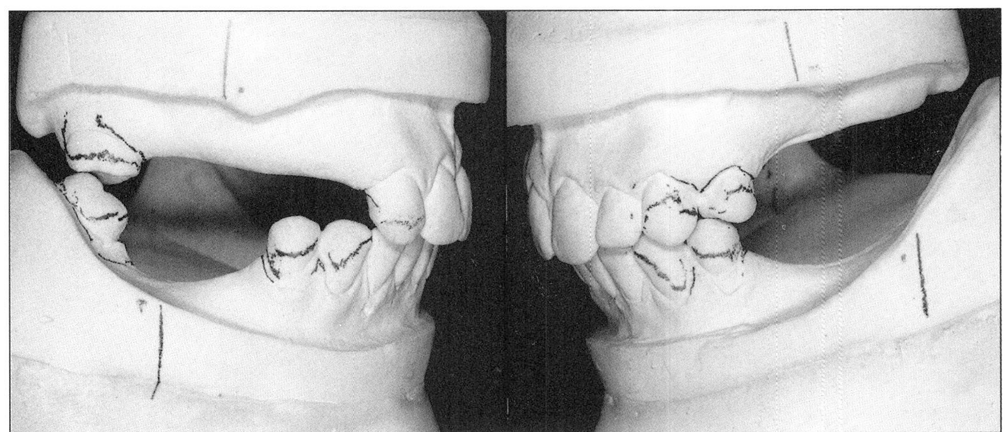

355

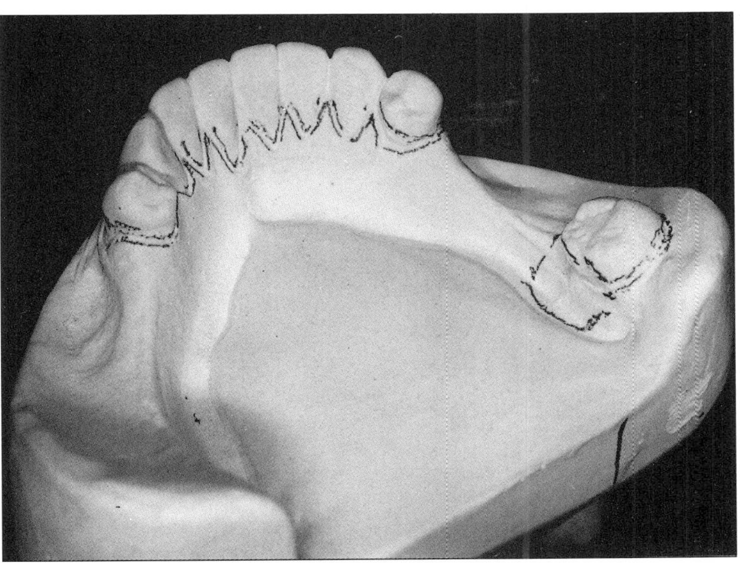

Incorrect design: patient no 2

Maxilla

- The survey line on 13 is very high. The entire retainer is therefore in undercut and the denture could not be inserted. The rigid shoulder of the retainer will not flex into an undercut.
- The 'horseshoe' connector finishes on the gingival margins. The connector is also too narrow for strength and the palatal aspect cuts across rugae instead of following their contour.
- The occlusal rest on 24 interferes with the only natural posterior occlusal stop on the left side.
- The undercut on the DB surface of 24 is too shallow for an I-bar (it should be moved to the mid-buccal surface). This appears to be a very small point, but it means the difference between effective or non-effective retention on the left side.
- The extension of denture stops short of the hamular notch on the left side and is thus losing valuable tissue support.

Mandible

- The survey line on 48 is high on the MB surface and low on the DB surface. Without tooth modification, the first (rigid) section of the retainer on 48 is therefore below the survey line. The flexible tip is above the survey line. The marked lingual tilt would not allow for a rigid reciprocating arm on the lingual surface without excessive tooth modification.
- 34 has no undercut on the DB surface. The I-bar onto this area is therefore not effective.
- The incisal rest on 32 and 31 is in an ideal position to act as indirect retention (the right-angled bisector of the fulcrum is between 34 and 48). However, it would be unaesthetic, interfere with the occlusion, and be irritating to the tongue. It is better to sacrifice the ideal position in such a case. Indirect retention can be achieved by an extension on to the cingulum of 43 (see design for patient no. 2, page 71).
- The occlusal rest on 34(D) interferes with the occlusion.
- The combination of the distal occlusal rest and I-bar on the DB surface will not stabilise the DEB against distal movement.

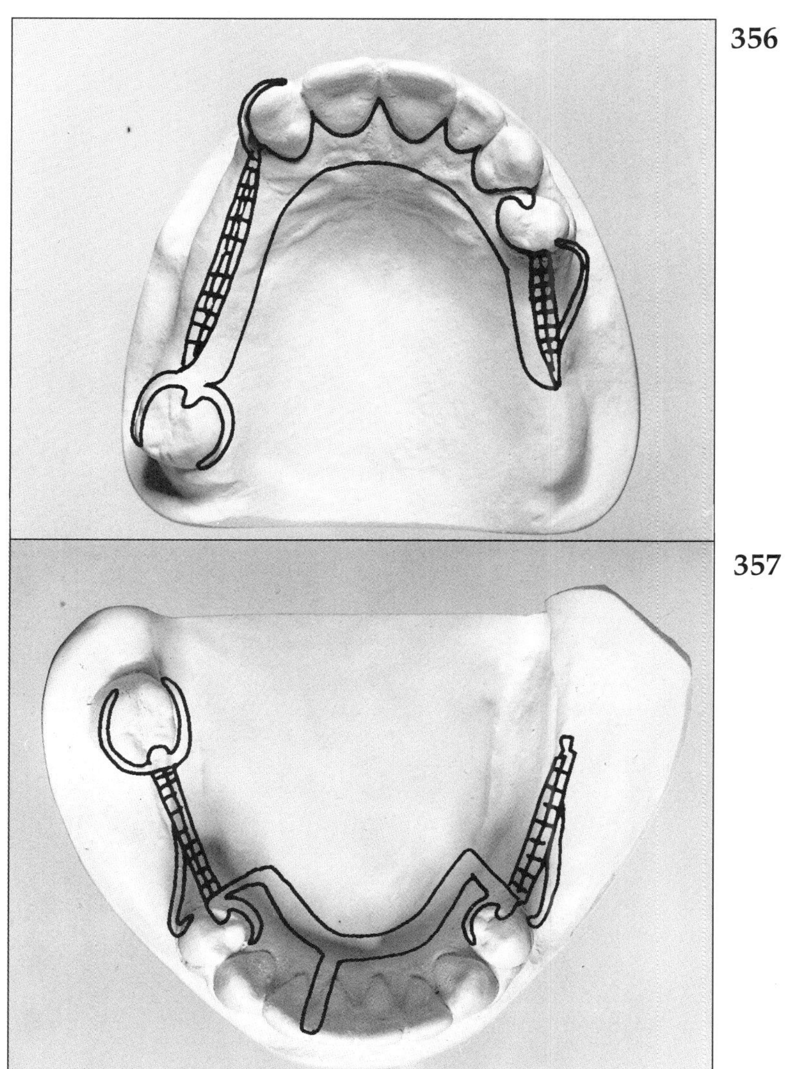

356

357

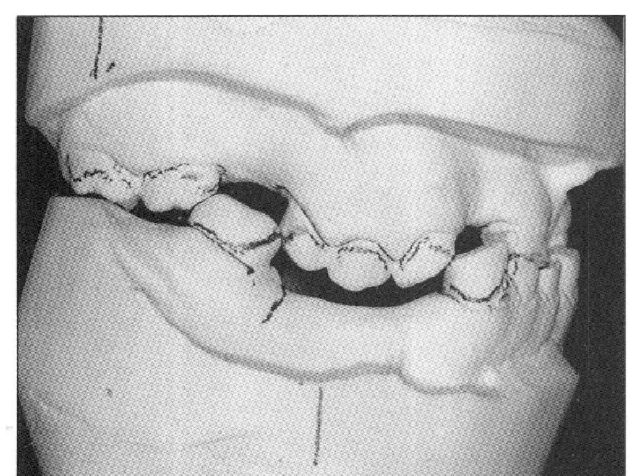
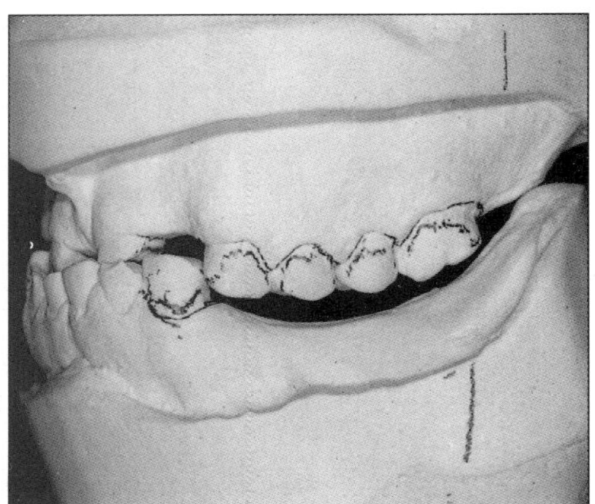

358   359

Incorrect design patient no 12

Maxilla

- The retentive triangle is very small. To be effective, it should be enlarged by extending the denture along the arch to 26.
- There are no undercuts on 17(DB), 14(MB) and 24(DB). The retainer tips on 17, 14 and 24 are therefore not effective.
- There are undercuts on 17(MB) and 24(MB). Without tooth modification, the rigid shoulders of the retainers on 17 and 24 are therefore in undercuts.
- There is no reciprocation for retainers on 17 and 24.
- The connector cuts straight across the rugae. It will also be clearly visible in the diastema between 11 and 21.
- There is no special acrylic anchorage, for example, posts and backing, for the isolated teeth to be replaced.

Mandible

- The DEB distal to 47 is contraindicated:
  it complicates the denture unnecessarily, making it less comfortable and therefore less likely to be worn;
  there is no space for it since these designs have not increased the OVD;
  it is unlikely to stop overeruption of 17 and 18.
- Both occlusal rests on 47 interfere with the occlusion.
- The survey line on 47 is high on the MB surface and low on the DB surface. Without tooth modification, the first (rigid) section of the retainer on 47 is therefore below the survey line. The flexible tip is above the survey line.
- There is no undercut on 43(DB). The I-bar on 43 is therefore not effective.
- The I-bar on 33(DB) will not prevent distal movement of the DEB without a mesial component.
- The lingual plate will show between 31 and 41.

Most important error

The designs have not addressed the patient's main complaint, i.e. the dentures do not restore OVD and the appearance of upper anteriors will not be improved.

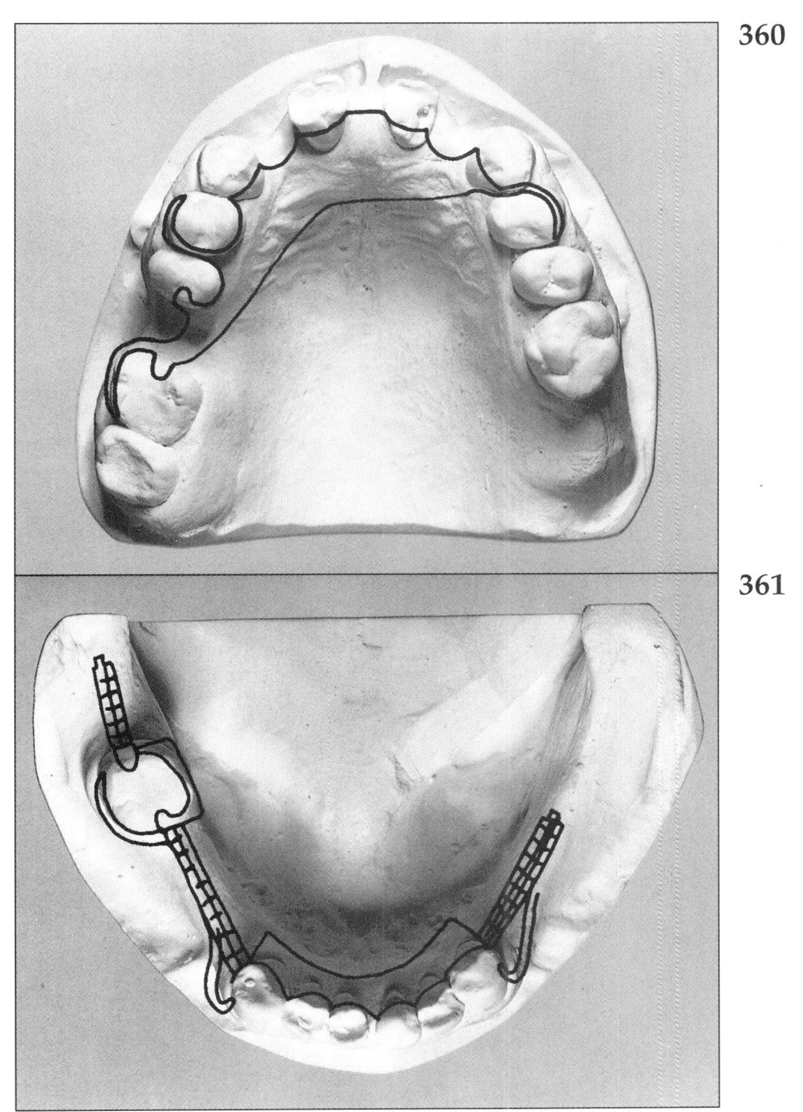

Bibliography

Academy of Denture Prosthetics, 'Principles, concepts and practices in prosthodontics'. *J Prosthet Dent*, 1989; **61**: 96–100.

Addy, M., Bates, J.F., 'The effect of partial dentures and chlorhexidine gluconate gel on plaque accumulation in the absence of oral hygiene'. *J Clin Periodontol*, 1977; **4**: 41–7.

Ahmad, I., Waters, N.E., 'Value of guide planes in denture retention'. *J Dent*, 1992; **20**: 59–64.

Anderson J.N., Bates, J.F., 'Cobalt-chromium partial dentures. A clinical survey'. *Br Dent J*, 1959; **107**: 57–62.

Anderson, J.N., Lammie, G.A., 'A clinical survey of partial dentures'. *Br Dent J*, 1952; **92**: 59–67.

Applegate, O.C., 'The cast saddle partial denture'. *J Am Dent Assoc and Den Cosmos*, 1937; **24**: 1280–91.

Axinn, S., 'Preparation of retentive areas of clasps in enamel'. *J Pros Dent*, 1975; **34**: 405–7.

Barco, M.T., Flinton, R.J., 'An overview of four partial denture clasps'. *Int J Prosthodont*, 1988; **1**: 159–64.

Basker, R.M., Harrison, A., Davenport, J.C., Marshall, J.L., 'Partial denture design in general dental practice – 10 years on'. *Br Dent J*, 1988; **165**: 245–9.

Basker, R.M., Tryde, G., 'Connectors for the mandibular partial denture: use of the sublingual bar'. *J Oral Rehabil*, 1977; **4**: 389–94.

Bates, J.F., 'Retention of partial dentures'. *Br Dent J*, 1980; **149**: 171–4.

Bates, J.F., Huggett, R., Stafford, G.D., *Removable Partial Denture Construction*, 3rd edn, Chapter 12, Butterworth, London, 1991.

Beckett, L.S., 'Influence of saddle classification on the design of partial removable restorations'. *J Prosthet Dent*, 1953; **3**: 506–16.

Beckett, L.S., 'Accurate occlusal relations in partial denture construction'. *J Prosthet Dent*, 1954; **4**: 487–95.

Berg, E., 'Periodontal problems associated with the use of distal extension partial dentures – a matter of construction?' *J Oral Rehabil*, 1985; **12**: 369–79.

Bergman, B., Hugoson, A., Olsson, C.O., 'Caries, periodontal and prosthetic findings in patients with removable partial dentures: a ten year longitudinal study'. *J Prosthet Dent*, 1982; **48**: 506–14.

Bissada, N.F., Ibraham, S.T., Barsoun, W.M., 'Gingival response to various types of removable partial dentures'. *J Periodontol*, 1974; 45: 651–9.

Brill, N., Tryde, G., Stoltze, K., El Ghamrawy, E.A., 'Ecologic changes in the oral cavity caused by removable partial dentures'. *J Prosthet Dent*, 1977; **38**: 138–48.

Campbell, L.D., 'Subjective reaction to major connector design for removable partial dentures'. *J Prosthet Dent*, 1977; **37**: 507–16.

Carlsson, G.E., Hedegard, B., Koivumaa, K.K., 'Studies in partial prostheses'. *Acta Odont Scand*, 1962; **20**: 95–119.

Carlsson, G.E., Hedegard, B., Koivumaa, K.K., 'Studies in partial prostheses'. *Acta Odont Scand*, 1965; **23**: 443–72.

Cotmore, J.M., Mingledorf, E.B., Pomerantz, J.M., Grasso, J.E., 'Removable partial denture survey: clinical practice today'. *J Prosthet Dent*, 1983; **49**: 321–7.

Cristadou, L., Osborne, J., Chamberlaine, J.B., 'The effect of partial denture design on the mobility of abutment teeth'. *Br Dent J*, 1973; **135**: 9–18.

Davenport, J.C., Basker, R.M., Heath, J.R., Ralph, J.P., *A Colour Atlas of Removable Partial Dentures*, Wolfe Medical, London, 1988.

Derry, A., Bertram, V., 'A clinical survey of removable partial dentures after 2 years usage'. *Acta Odont Scand*, 1970; **28**: 581–98.

De Van, M.M., 'The nature of the partial denture foundation: suggestions for its preservation'. *J Prosthet Dent*, 1952; **2**: 210–18.

Dixon, D.L., Breeding, L.C., Swift, E.J., 'Use of partial coverage porcelain laminate to enhance clasp retention'. *J Prosthet Dent*, 1990; **63**: 55–8.

El-Ghamrawy., 'Quantitative changes in dental plaque formation related to removable partial dentures . *J Oral Rehabil*, 1967; **3**: 116–20.

Farrell, J.H., 'Partial denture tolerance'. *Dent Practit,* 1969; **19**: 162–4.

Frantz, W.R., 'Variations in a removable maxillary partial denture design by dentists'. *J Prosthet Dent,* 1975; **34**: 625–33.

Freilich, M.A., Breeding, L.C., Keagle, J.G., Garnick, J.J., 'Fixed partial dentures supported by periodontally compromised teeth'. *J Prosthet Dent,* 1991; **65**: 607–11.

Gaston, G.W., 'Rest area preparation for removable partial dentures'. *J Prosthet Dent* 1960; **10**: 124–34.

Graham, C.H., Beckett, L.S., 'Partial denture design – a group project'. *Aust Pros Soc Bull,* 1986; **16**: 71–7.

Hobkirk, J.A., Strahan, J.D., 'The influence on the gingival tissues of prostheses incorporating gingival relief areas'. *J Dent,* 1979; **7**: 15–21.

Holmes, J.G., 'The altered cast impression procedure for the distal extension removable partial denture'. *Dent Clin North America,* 1970; **14**: 569–82.

Ibbetson, R.J., Setchell, D.J., 'Treatment of the worn dentition'. *Dent Update,* 1989; **16**: 247, 250–3, 300–2, 305–7.

Jacobson, T.E., Krol, A.J., 'Rotational path removable partial denture design'. *J Prosthet Dent,* 1982; **48**: 370–6.

Jenkins, C.B.G., Berry, D.C., 'Modification of tooth contours by acid etch retained resin for prosthetic purposes'. *Br Dent J,* 1976; **14**: 89–90.

Jung, T., 'The reaction of gingival tissues to removable partial dentures'. *Proc Eur Prosth Assoc,* 1980: 38–42.

King, G.E., 'Dual path design for removable partial dentures'. *J Prosthet Dent,* 1978; **39**: 392–95.

Koivumaa, K.K., 'Changes in periodontal tissues and supporting structures connected with partial dentures'. *Dent Abs,* 1957; **2**: 468–9.

Kratochvil, F.J., 'Influence of occlusal rest position and clasp design on movement of abutment teeth'. *J Prosthet Dent,* 1963; **13**: 114–24.

Kratochvil, F.J., 'Maintaining supporting structures with removable partial dentures'. *J Prosthet Dent,* 1971; **25**: 167–74.

Kratochvil, F.J., Leupold, R.J., 'An altered cast procedure to improve tissue support for removable partial dentures'. *J Prosthet Dent,* 1965; **15**: 672–8.

Krol, A.J., 'Clasp design for extension base removable partial dentures'. *J Prosthet Dent,* 1973; **29**: 408–15.

Krol, A.J., Finzen, F.C., 'Rotational path removable partial dentures. Part 1. Replacement of posterior teeth. Part 2. Replacement of anterior teeth'. *Int J Prosthodont,* 1988; **1**: 17–27; 135–42.

Krol, A.J., Jacobson, T.E., Finzen, F.C., *Removable Partial Denture Design Outline Syllabus,* 4th edn, San Rafael, California, 1990.

Lammie, G.A., Laird, W.R.E., *Partial Dentures (Osborne and Lammie),* 5th edn, Blackwell, Oxford, 1986.

Lechner, S.K., 'A longitudinal survey of removable partial dentures I. Patient assessment of dentures'. *Aust Dent J,* 1985*a*; **30**: 112–17.

Lechner, S.K., 'A longitudinal survey of removable partial dentures II. Tissue reactions to various denture components'. *Aust Dent J,* 1985*b*; **30**: 291–5.

Lechner, S.K., 'The distal extension saddle partial denture: a review'. *Aust Prosthet J,* 1987; **1**: 59–64.

McDermott, I. G., Esposito, S., 'The cingulum bar major connector'. *Gen Dent,* 1983; **31**: 292–3.

McGivney, G.P., Castleberry, D.J., *McCracken's Removable Partial Prosthodontics,* 8th edn, Chapter 7, Mosby, St Louis, 1989.

MacGregor, A.R., 'Stress-breaking in partial dentures'. *Aust Pros Soc Bull,* 1986; **16**: 65–70.

MacGregor, A.R., *Fenn, Liddelow & Gimson's Clinical Dental Prosthetics,* 3rd edn, Butterworth, London, 1989.

MacGregor, A.R., Miller, T.P.G., Farah, J.W., 'The support of bounded saddles'. *J Dent* 1983; **11**: 139–50.

McKinstry, R.E., Minsley, G.E., Wood, M.T., 'The effect of clinical experience on dental students' ability to design removable partial denture frameworks'. *J Prosthet Dent,* 1989; **62**: 563–6.

Mahonen, K.T., Virtanen, K.K., 'An alternative treatment for excessive tooth wear. A clinical report'. *J Prosthet Dent,* 1991; **65**: 463–5.

Meeuwissen. R., Keltjens, H.M., Battistuzzi, P.G., 'Cingulum bars as a major connector for mandibular removable partial dentures'. *J Prosthet Dent,* 1991; **66**: 221–3.

Miller, E. L., Grasso, J.E., *Removable Partial Prosthodontics*, 2nd edn, Chapter 6, Williams and Wilkins, Baltimore, 1981.

Neill, D.J., Walter, J.D., *Partial Dentures*, 2nd edn, Blackwell, Oxford, 1983.

Owall, B.E., Taylor, R. L., 'A survey of dentitions and removable partial dentures constructed for patients in North America'. *J Prosthet Dent*, 1989; **61**: 465–70.

Roach, F.E., 'Mouth survey and design of partial dentures'. *J Am Dent Assoc*, 1934; **21**: 1166–76.

Schiesser, F.J., 'The neutral zone and polished surface in complete dentures'. *J Prosthet Dent*, 1964; **14**: 856–65.

Schwalm, C.A., Smith, D.E., Erichson, J.A., 'A clinical study of patients 1 and 2 years after placement of removable partial dentures. *J Prosthet Dent*, 1977; **38**: 380–91.

Schwarz, W.D., Barsby, M.J., 'Tooth alteration procedures prior to partial denture construction'. *Dent Update*, 1984; **11**: 234–7.

Seemann, S.K. (Lechner, S.K.), 'A study of the relationship between periodontal disease and the wearing of partial dentures'. *Aust Dent J*, 1963; **8**: 206–8.

Smith, B.G., 'Toothwear: aetiology and diagnosis'. *Dent Update*, 1989; **16**: 204–12.

Stillwell, C., 'Sublingual bars: prescription and technique'. *Quintessence Int*, 1988; **19**: 555–8.

Stipho, H.K.D., Murphy, W.M., Adams, D., 'Effect of oral prostheses on plaque accumulation'. *Br Dent J*, 1979; **145**: 47–50.

Taylor, R.L., Reese, R., *Removable Partial Denture Restoration: Function and Aesthetics*, 1984, pp 5–47. Austenal Products Laboratory, Howmedica, Inc, Chicago.

Thomas, C.J., de Kok, M., 'A clinical study of the modified Equipoise clasp'. *Aust Prosthet J*, 1990; **4**: 53–7.

Tjan, A.H.L., Miller, G.D., 'Some esthetic factors in a smile'. *Prosthet Dent*, 1984; **51**: 24–8.

Tomlin, H.R., Osborne, J., 'Cobalt-chromium partial dentures: a clinical survey'. *Br Dent J*, 1961; **110**: 307–10.

Trushkowsky, R., Bahman, G., 'Restoration of occlusal vertical dimension by means of a silica-coated onlay removable partial denture in conjunction with dentin bonding. A clinical report'. *J Prosthet Dent*, 1991; **66**: 283–6.

Tuominen, R., Ranta, K., Paunio, I., 'Wearing of removable partial dentures in relation to periodontal pockets'. *J Oral Rehabil*, 1989; **16**: 119–26.

Wagner, A.G., Traweek, F.C., 'A comparison of major connectors for removable partial dentures'. *J Prosthet Dent*, 1982; **47**: 242–5.

Walter, J.D., 'The 1988 partial denture survey'. *Proc Brit Soc Study Prosthet Dent*, 1989: 30.

Walter, J.D., *Removable Partial Denture Design*, 2nd edn, Chapter 6, British Dental Association, London, 1990.

Watt, D.M., MacGregor, A.R., *Designing Partial Dentures*, Wright, Bristol, 1984.

Wetherall, J.D., Smales, R.J., 'Partial denture failures; a long term clinical study'. *J Dent*, 1980; **8**: 333–40.

Williams, D.R., 'A rationale for the management of advanced tooth wear'. *J Oral Rehabil*, 1987; **14**: 77–89.

Witter, D.J., Elteren, P. van, Kayser, A. F., Rossum, M.J. M. van, 'The effect of removable partial dentures in the oral function in shortened dental arches'. *J Oral Rehabil*, 1989; **16**: 27–33.

Witter, D.J., Elteren, P. van, Kayser, A.F., Rossum, M.J.M. van, 'Oral comfort in shortened dental arches'. *J Oral Rehabil*, 1990; **17**: 137–43.

Wright, W., 'Abutment tooth modification for removable partial denture therapy'. *Compendium*, 1989; **10**: 40–7.

Index